Healing Without Lifting a Finger

Alex Cochran

DISCLAIMER:

The author of this book is not a medical practitioner. This book does not give medical advice. Any method and theory of healing presented in this book is meant for information sharing purposes only. The information presented in this book is not meant for any medical consumer. It does not replace medical advice or treatment by your physician, and not made to replace your existing effective healing solutions. Consult other experts and medical consultants in their field when deciding on your best medical treatment options. Therefore, the author and the publisher assume no responsibility for any person's interpretation or use of the information in this book.

CONTENTS

Foreword

ADDITIONAL NOTES FOR EACH METHOD

FOREWORD

I experienced the benefit of realizing that there's such a thing as "healing without lifting a finger". And when I put to use what I found, its usefulness and effectiveness became apparent. Gradually, the conclusion became simple. No true physical and bodily health can be obtained without first experiencing that sense of healing in one's mind and one's thinking. I saw that any healing is impossible without one's own spiritual self in the process of healing. Answers come eventually as the reason for any physical illness, or problem, is spiritual.

By the end of 2012 I had enough experience to be fully convinced that the methods you're about to review in this book are real. I used them on regular basis and I wanted to share them with others. I had a clear enough idea of how the methods worked and used them in my daily life. Sometimes in combination with other methods, and sometimes individually, or in groups with like-minded people. I used them in my own way and experienced their effectiveness in a way that made sense. All this, of course, is different from writing a book to make it very easy to share with other people. To do so, I needed more than my personal step-by-step outline of each method. Each step of each healing method would need to be shared in a way that would make a sometimes difficult subject of *healing* relatable to people with their own health experiences and unique beliefs.

A change of mind came as I drove early morning in my

Washington, DC, neighborhood on Valentine's Day 2013, my wish to share my methods with others returned in a form of a title: *Healing Without Lifting a Finger*. I finally felt what it represented to me. However, this answer was quickly replaced by more questions. Could my wish to share *healing without lifting a finger* methods mean that I'd be willing to try to explain a very complex subject? Should I make my collection of methods into a community service project? Or, share about the hope of healing with people who wanted to achieve their desired level of health? While like questions were inspiring, I wanted clear answers.

In no time I put the *healing without lifting a finger* methods into a book and even included generous, lecture-like explanations to go along. I needed advice about how to actually share the knowledge with other people and in a way that could be applied. Dolores Cannon made a positive impression on the book you're about to read. I think that Dolores really wanted to share helpful information with her readers. From her Ozark Mountain publishing she sent back an informative letter in which she explained how the explanations for each method needed to improve. The difficult, and often misunderstood subject needed to be simplified to be helpful. It was clear, readers only want clear and simple steps in each method. It was a sad day for *healing without lifting a finger* when I found that Dolores would not be there to look over the improvements. On October 2014 she transitioned back to the spirit world. Her personal return letter contributed to the book. The steps are easy and simple to follow. And also, for readers like me, who like reading more background explanations behind each method, there is also an additional section with more details and explanations.

I continue sharing *healing without lifting a finger* methods with others. It is a subject I enjoy to continuously explore and apply daily. With gained experience, I became even more convinced that *healing without lifting a finger* is absolutely possible. Absolutely valid. And in some cases, where conventional medicine is unable to give answers, these and like methods can inspire you to continue achieving your ultimately desired level of health. This is the message I wanted to share: healing doesn't have to stop and can always continue to take place. The people can achieve their desired level of health.

The true essence of healing is so much more than body, or even the mind. Isn't it simply another way of saying development, growth and improvement? We can all develop on so many levels and there's no limit to the potential.

It's now 2020, and it's been six years since I first shared *Healing Without Lifting a Finger* with readers, I continue to be convinced by the effectiveness of the presented methods. And I think it's just an edge of the inspiring journey I simply call *healing without lifting a finger*.

INTRODUCTION

It's totally obvious that we are so much more than simply the physical bodies we inhabit. We are immortal spiritual beings with boundless possibilities. Even though that's all we think sometimes, our bodies are just a very tiny portion of who we are. We are simply too infinite to have the true source of our physical illness be physical.

As we go on as this civilization we find that healing someone's physical body without addressing their spiritual needs is not going to last. We find that we must be more involved in our whole healing process. We must allow us to heal ourselves and to discover alternative ways to do this. We must realize that in addition to our conventional medicine, there are also very effective healing alternatives out there. Some of them invite our infinite potential and resourcefulness to be involved.

And, yes, we must realize that the key to lasting physical healing is not always found in toxic drugs, harassment by invasive surgeries, or wasted treasure. Sometimes, healing is not about bothering our bodies, but bothering to use our own consciousness.

My own journey to get a better understanding of how our consciousness can be used for healing took me to the discovery of the 27 methods in this book. Some of the methods came from my upbringing. Others came from my friends who've shared them with me. Other methods started from seeing the same points made in various books from past to present thinkers. And others came from what I think maybe past experiences when this sort of knowledge was more common.

As I used these methods, I became thoroughly convinced that conscious healing methods are the most important source of physical health. And that they must be shared with others because it's just too big of a subject for one person to have. I'm not sure what someone else in a similar position would have called these types of methods, but in my mind I simply referred to them as 'healing without lifting a finger'. Likewise, I tried to come up with a simple name for each of the methods.

As years went by I decided to do what I could to share these views. One thing that emerged again and again on this journey is that healing is a free thing and truly anyone can have it. Healing is in the frame of mind and how we see the reality around us, and also how we choose to construct our reality. The alternate reality that I discovered for myself is that our ability to heal without lifting a finger is a totally natural thing. This ability is not even so much a gift to us. It's a given before we lose our awareness and get in the way of our own spiritual development.

Chapter 1

THE FIRST THOUGHT OF THE DAY

The Background

Usually, in the time right before you fully wake up is when your mind is at its freshest and receptive. This is why what you say to yourself at this point will matter for the rest of the day. The ideas will literally plant themselves in your head.

If you want to achieve healing then this particular time of day for you will be beneficial if you will put this time to a good use. If, during this suggestive time, you reinforce your self-suggestions that you're unwell and that you're not healing, then your body will use your suggestion to continue down the same path. If, however, you say to yourself that you're feeling better. And then further reinforce your first waking-up statement with <u>seeing</u>, <u>feeling</u> and <u>sensing in every way possible</u> what it is you want to achieve, then your body will use that suggestion to bring you closer to the level of healing you desire. Where your thought is, there your healing will be also.

Step 1

Learn to regard your waking up process as a very sacred and important time. It impacts not only the rest of your day, but also the overall healing you will accomplish for the rest of the day.

(Hint: Take this time to prepare yourself and your mind for

the next morning you're going to wake up. What will be the first thoughts that will cross your mind when you wake up? Don't procrastinate, but begin to think about some of the things which you expect will come to mind on that important morning occasion. Contemplate some of the changes you'll make in your overall waking routine.)

(Hint: Start getting used to waking up with only the thoughts you want. Are you one of those who are in the habit of tallying up all the aches and pains every time you shift your foot out of bed? If so, then this is the time to prepare to change that.)

Step 2

Come up with just the kind of statement that would best sum up the achievement of your desired level of health.

(Hint: Exclude from that statement anything and everything that doesn't happen to match your ultimate health goal. The easiest way to do this is to focus on coming up with the type of statement that is the polar opposite of what you do not want. For example, if you know you always typically start out your day with a certain ache or symptom, then come up with the statement that is the opposite of that.)

(Hint: Having a clear idea of the healing you need will make your desired statement much easier to figure out.)

Step 3

Now, as soon as you wake up <u>see</u>, <u>feel</u> and <u>sense in every way possible</u> your healing taking place.

(Hint: It might take you a couple of mornings to get the hang of it.)

Last Step

If you put your mind to it, you will quickly get in the habit of only focusing on the achievement of your desired level of health as your first thought of the day. If you have, you will see, sense, and feel in every way possible that you're coming to the achievement of your desired level of health. Keep it up!

Chapter 2

LETTING GO OF ANGER

The Background

Anger is debilitating and counterproductive to healing. Healing is not about holding on to anger. And anger is not the same as healing. Anger is a negative thought, while healing is positive. Healing is about a positive frame of mind, and about giving yourself every possible chance to enter into the positive frame of mind.

Our frame of mind is made up of many thoughts. These thoughts have their own unique vibration. Some thoughts have a negative vibration and some have positive. When our frame of mind is made up of negative vibrations it is said that our frame of mind has a lower vibration. Conversely, if our frame of mind is made up of positive vibrations it is said that our frame of mind has a higher vibration.

When we allow ourselves to receive the thoughts of the like vibration they in turn set the vibration of our frame of mind. And when our frame of mind resonates at a particular vibration it in turn sets the overall vibration of our physical bodies. So that ultimately, our thoughts, mind and body operate at the same vibration. We find this is reflected in overall performance of our physical bodies. This means that if we allow ourselves to be dominated by thoughts of anger, our overall physical vibration will lower to a negative level. Clearly, this is not something anyone wants when they try to create a positive healing vibration.

Step 1

Whenever you feel angry or upset try to get in the habit of simply acknowledging to yourself in real time that that is what's going on. Bring those thoughts from the background and into the foreground of your awareness.

(Hint: Do not lose your awareness of the instances when you get angry or resentful.)

Step 2

Now explore some of the patterns associated with that anger or resentment. Developing a habit of noticing when you get angry or resentful will help you explore the reasons that cause you to be angry or upset.

(Hint: Some of the questions you might want to ask yourself here are: 'How often do I get angry?', 'Do I always get angry at around the same time or for the same reasons?', 'What is it about that particular situation that causes me to respond in such a way, or to be angry?')

Step 3

Look to see if the causes or reasons for your anger can be removed. Be creative and put your thinking cap on. Ask yourself, 'Is keeping my anger worth the healing it prevents me from achieving?'

(Hint: If your circumstances are harsh and will not allow you to get rid of the causes of anger right away, then simply continue to monitor your levels of anger and their reasons.

Likewise, take comfort in knowing that no matter how depressing those causes may be, they are always temporary if dealt with in a proactive way.)

Step 4

Look back onto your life, as far back as you're comfortable, and see if there is anything there that still causes you to feel angry or resentful.

(Hint: The question you might want to ask yourself here might go something like this, 'Does the following event or situation from my past still cause me to feel angry or resentful about what happened?' If the answer is yes, then look into ways of resolving it.)

Last Step

Explore all the things that are opposite of anger and resentment, such as for example, increasing joy, happiness and satisfaction in your life. Go ahead, give yourself a break, do more of what you enjoy, more of the things that satisfy. In the process you might just discover that this will serve as an ironclad antidote for whatever it is your life might bring your way.

Chapter 3

FREEDOM FROM IMBALANCE AND DEATH IDEAS

The Background

Human life offers a lot of stimuli to focus and concentrate on. These stimuli constantly compete for our attention. Some stimuli we automatically accept and some we automatically repel. Whether a particular stimulus is repelled or rejected is determined by whether or not it appeals to our frame of mind. In very basic terms, if a stimulus matches the vibration of our frame of mind it is accepted, if not it is repelled. Another simple way to think of this process is that every stimulus is a type of thought form, and to think of our frame of mind as the place where those thoughts can be processed.

Our frame of mind is made up of many like thought forms which basically match in vibration. When our frame of mind is formed with those thoughts it then tells our physical body what to do. So that ultimately, our thoughts, mind and body reach the same vibration. The thoughts of illness or death also have their particular vibration that is either accepted or repelled by our frame of mind. For example, if you're very young and healthy, then that is your frame of mind and it is very easy to repel the ideas of illness or death. This is because the thought vibrations of death and illness are incompatible. However, when someone is mentally upset, their vibration is lowered and the lower thoughts of illness and death become acceptable.

Our particular frame of mind is based on our choice. And we can choose what thoughts to accept and which to reject based on our frame of mind. When we choose to raise the vibration of our frame of mind, then that creates a framework to receive the like thoughts of higher vibration. So that by raising the vibration of our frame of mind with the thoughts of healing and rejuvenation, our physical body's vibration is then raised to that level as well. Those thoughts become our reality. On the other hand, if we choose to nourish our frame of mind only with the thoughts of illness and dying, then it will be reflected in our chosen frame of mind, which will then influence how our bodies will end up feeling. This is because like attracts like.

Step 1

Ask yourself whether or not you have any ideas of having any imbalance, or illness, in your body and mind. Ask yourself whether or not you think you're dying.

(Hint: It doesn't matter if that death is a year, years, or many decades from now. Try to be as honest this time as you possibly can.)

Step 2

Convert the ideas you have into their polar opposites. For example, every time you think you're imbalanced, or ill, or might have it, do your best to think balance, health, etc.

(Hint: Focus only on your optimally desired level of health and at the exclusion of anything and everything that doesn't happen to match that desire. For example, every time you think you're dying or will die, do your best to think, life, revitalization, rejuvenation, etc. Be as specific as you can.)

Step 3

See all of the illnesses, or death ideas from your past life in your mind. Perhaps, it's seeing your grandmother age, or perhaps it's something somebody told you on the schoolyard when they explained to you the difference between a natural death and murder. Now, go back to those situations and see them in the new light by converting those words.

(Hint: It's not about denial that those things exist, or that certain 'hereditary' factors predispose you to some illness. You're simply addressing those profound situations from the new, more informed point of view. More applicably, you're dealing with those ideas face to face so that you can be free from them to go on achieving your optimally desired level of health.)

Last Step

Continue to take regular 'mental cleanses' from those ideas, because so long as you're free from them, they are powerless to stop you from coming closer to your achievement of your optimally desired level of health.

(Hint: Even though our society purports to espouse to health and life, at its present state it bursts with ideas of imbalance and death. These ideas are very subtle, and sometimes entertaining. When one is not aware of this, they can enter one's thinking just like that.)

Chapter 4

LETTING GO OF FEAR

The Background

Fear is probably the most powerful negative thought a human can have. When someone is afraid it becomes much harder to function and feel free to do what one truly wishes. If your pursuit is to achieve healing, then fear of an illness is not the best mate to have on your journey.

A state of fear also influences our frame of mind, and it in turn, dictates how our bodies respond. When we're afraid, our heart rate increases, we sweat and become jittery. Our fears also dictate how we think. When we have thoughts of fear, we tense up and it becomes harder for our mind to focus and concentrate only on the healing we want. It becomes harder to relax and let the healing energy to freely flow and access our bodies. In short, when we're afraid, we close up on several levels. And when we close off, we shut ourselves off to our healing potential. We don't want to go out and explore. We just want to close ourselves up in our fort until the weather passes.

Probably the easiest way to think of fear is that it is a negative (lower) vibration. Healing, on the other hand, is a positive vibration. So that when someone desires healing but has fear, they create a dissonance in their thinking. It becomes like a tug of war between the negative thinking and the positive thinking until ultimately either a positive or a negative vibration prevails. This means that if a person wants the positive healing to take place in their body, then they must make their frame of mind more conducive to accept more of the positive thoughts, while at the same time work on reducing the negative thoughts. And fear is a negative thought that can be resolved if a person chooses to have a different frame of mind.

Step 1

Briefly look around yourself for the first fear that jumps to mind, no matter how small or big it may be. Select a particular fear you want to work with.

(Hint: Smaller is easier to deal with and to use for practice. For example, perhaps you had a fear of missing the bus to work. Maybe being late or missing your lunch. When you've picked a fear, or a couple of those small fears to deal with, we're ready for the next step.)

Step 2

Bring your attention to your fear and try to understand where it's coming from.

(Hint: The questions you might want to ask yourself here might sound like this: 'How long have I had this particular fear?', 'Why do I have this fear?', or 'What events cause me to experience it?')

Step 3

Ask yourself if there's anything you can do to resolve the situation or an event in your life which causes your particular fear.

(Hint: Take all the time that you need. This is not a competition. Rest assured that every little fear you let go of from your life means absolutely that you're coming closer to your achievement of your optimally desired level of health. Because letting go of every fear, no matter how small, counts.)

Step 4

Shift your attention to your past experiences, years or decades back, all the way back to childhood.

(Hint: The questions to ask here might be, 'Was there anything I was particularly afraid of when I was a child?' or 'What was the first major, or significant fear I had when I was a child?' Perhaps it was an unjustified fear of water, so much so that you were afraid to get aboard any ship even if it was docked, or wouldn't go to the public pool. Or, perhaps you were afraid of a certain person, personality, a physical type, etc. Or, maybe even an animal. Or, whatever it was that made you afraid. As you do so, ask yourself whether or not you're still afraid of those things, or if you've been able to overcome your fear and how.)

Last Step

Continue to be vigilant for any sign of fear. Fear has a subtle way of creeping in on people, especially when they least expect it.

(Hint: Use your fearlessness to your advantage, especially,

when it comes to exploring other areas of your life, and areas of opportunity.)

Chapter 5

RESOLVING PAIN
(*WITH ADDITIONAL METHOD*)

The Background

Physical pain is perhaps the strongest human attention-getting signal. It is a signal that there's a high priority message that a person needs to pay attention to and respond to right away. This message process basically involves two parties, the sender and the recipient. The sender is a person's own higher self (aka higher consciousness/spirit) who's signaling that they are sending a very important message. And the recipient is a person who's noticing the signal of the arrival of a high priority message from their higher self. It is also important to keep in mind that the message that your higher self has for you is always benevolent. It is meant to help you evolve and get on with your journey. It is always in your best interest, and that of others

The degree of pain a person notices during this message process gives a pretty accurate indication of the scale of priority that their message has. The messages with the higher priority are therefore usually accompanied by the greater attention-getting signals. If the message behind the physical signal (pain) gets ignored, it often increases. And this is what the pain is apparently designed to do. Conversely, if a person gets the signal and receives their message then the pain had served its purpose. If not, then a person's higher self will use additional signals until they ring through and a person gets their message.

Each message is personal and in some way appropriate to its recipient. The message is also very literal to each recipient. This means that once the recipient is able to notice the signal and pick up the message, it will be readily understood by them on a personal level. They will have the moment of recognition, which will let them know that the message was correct for them. This whole message process also involves cooperation of the parts of the physical body. And every part of the body that's involved in sending the pain signal gives an indication of what the message is about. This makes every part of the body that's involved appropriate to the kind of message that's being sent from the higher self.

Once the message is received, the recipient can then find out what their message is telling them to do. And if it makes sense to them, find out how they can do what their higher self is telling them in the message. What should be kept in mind is that the higher self would not send a pain signal to a person unless there was something very important going on. And when it resorts to pain signal, chances are that something has gone amiss in the communication between the sender and the recipient. If the things have gotten this extreme, a person was not listening to the previous messages by their higher self.

Trying to ignore the pain signal in order to avoid having to deal with a personal message from their higher self does not help a person act in their best interest, and spiritual development. This response will cause the signal to get more drastic. The best way to get rid of pain (signal) is to find out its source (message) and figure out ways to do something about it. Even if the causes of physical pain are not readily apparent right away, a person should still try to figure out what it is their higher self is trying to tell them with their physical body. It's drawing their attention to something in their life that needs their urgent attention.

Step 1

If at some time you acknowledge that you're feeling pain (or irritation), you can understand that you're receiving the signal that your higher self has a high priority message for you.

(Hint: By choosing to move your thoughts from the signal and onto trying to figure out your message, the pain (irritation) thought in your mind will decrease. This will cause the overall vibration of your frame of mind to increase, and instruct your physical body and your frame of mind to operate at a lighter (more positive) thought vibration. This is a type of relief.)

(Hint: Save yourself the time and try to see if there's any way you can remove the cause of your pain (annoyance) from your life. If, once you remove that cause, you find that the pain (annoyance) goes away, then it means that you have successfully received and acted on the message you were supposed to receive.)

Step 2

Make a choice that you will receive the message that could be causing you to experience the pain (or annoyance) signal.

Step 3

Ask your higher self, higher consciousness, or spirit, or whatever term you're most comfortable with, what message it wants you to receive.

(Hint: Phrase it in any way you want, and through whatever medium you feel most comfortable with.)

(Hint: Beware, that the area of your body where you're experiencing pain (or annoyance) is a huge part of the message, and is often a clue of the message. This gives you a big part of the literal answer to the message already. More on this can be found in the Method 9) *Communication/Conversation with the affected area* and Method *12) Conversation with the Higher self/Higher consciousness on perceived lessons.*)

(Hint: Keep asking for as long as you need to receive your message. Your Higher Self is a higher you. This means that you have your divine right to communicate with it at your pleasure.)

(Hint: Be patient as you begin to receive the message. It may first come in parts. And understand that if you weren't ready to receive the message, it wouldn't have been sent.)

Step 4

When you acknowledge that you have received a message (or a first part of it) from your higher self, make sure you act responsibly. Figure out if the message is in your best interest (from your higher self), or not.

(Hint: You can tell that the message you received is from

your higher self if it is benevolent and tells you to do something in your best interest, as well as in the best interest of others.)

Step 5

Make a choice that you will do what your message tells you.

(Hint: Doing what your message tells you lets your higher self know that you are willing to cooperate, and the signal for this message can go away.)

Last Step

Find a way to do what your message is telling you to do. And if it's appropriate, do it.

(Hint: If you feel you need additional guidance about the most appropriate way to do what your message is telling you, feel free to ask your higher self (or your spirit guides, etc.) for additional assistance.)

(Hint: The message that your higher self has for you is always benevolent. It is meant to help you   develop and get on with your journey. It is always in your best interest, and that of others.)

Additional method:

RESOLVING THE KIND OF PAIN THAT'S A MANAGEABLE ANNOYANCE

Background

This is an effective method for resolving such things as minor and temporary pain (irritation). You can find the Background to this method in the last half of this book (*Additional notes for each method #5*).

Step 1

If you happen to acknowledge that you have a minor pain, temporary pain (irritation or annoyance) that you feel you need to ignore for a time, then begin to tell yourself in your mind anything that is the polar opposite of that feeling of pain, and at the exclusion of anything and everything that doesn't happen to match that goal.

(Hint: The opposite of pain is relief, comfort, soothing, etc. For example, if you feel in pain, then go ahead and just say the opposite of pain every time you happen to feel it. A statement to look for might go something like this, 'I'm feeling more and more relieved', or 'I actually feel more and more comfortable', or 'My body and mind are being soothed', etc. Keep saying this to yourself over and over again as long as it takes. Give it some effort and you will see the results, because pain is just a thought, and yes, like any thought it can be accepted or repelled.)

(Hint: Practice switching your heavy (negative) thoughts

with positive (lighter) thoughts as long as it takes you to become proficient at it.)

Step 2

Focus and <u>see</u>, <u>feel</u> and <u>sense in every way possible</u> only that thought which you want to see, feel and sense.

(Hint: When you practice this step, exclude anything and everything that doesn't happen to match only your desired thought. <u>Think</u>, <u>see</u> and <u>feel</u> only that feeling which you want to feel. Pain is just a thought. So if, for example, you've burned your finger, then think, see and feel coldness and soothing of that part of the body while you think to yourself comforting thoughts. Remember, polar opposite, or lighter (higher vibration) thoughts.)

Last Step

As you apply this method to a pain other than a minor irritation, make sure that you do not make it into a way of simply ignoring the messages from your higher self.

(Hint: If you are still supposed to receive your message, then your higher self will have the last word. And make sure you ultimately receive it.)

Chapter 6

BECOMING A LITTLE CHILD

The Background

What you think is what you are. When someone's a child they think like a child. When someone's old, they think like an old person. When someone's rejuvenating they have rejuvenating thoughts. And since rejuvenation and youth are usually synonymous with health, then we often think of our healing as becoming rejuvenated. While getting old we stereotype as the state of acquiring illnesses.

Your physical body has a particular vibration. This vibration didn't just come from nowhere. In basic terms, every solid object has its own particular vibration. This vibration is dictated by the frame of mind, and the thought forms that a person accepts or repels.

While living in the body, a person's frame of mind gradually changes based on the thoughts that a person has accepted throughout their life. This is because a person's frame of mind is made up of those thought forms which closely match its vibration level. For example, if a person gradually saw themselves as getting physically older, it means that their perceived aging was reflected by their particular thought forms. On other hand, if a person saw themselves as being physically rejuvenated, then it means their perceived youthfulness was reflected by their particular thought forms.

Step 1

See, feel, and sense yourself in every way possible becoming a little child; or, rather, being a little child.

(Hint: Begin by relaxing and trying to recall as best you can what it felt like to be a little child. As you recall that memory, do your best to see, feel and sense in every way possible what your body and mind actually felt like at the time.)

Last Step

Now, <u>see</u>, <u>feel</u>, and <u>sense in every way possible</u> how cell by cell, nerve ending by nerve ending, fiber by fiber, organ by organ, hair by hair, etc., your body becomes that of a little child.

(Hint: Your cells always rejuvenate and regenerate anyways, so, all you have to do is simply see, feel and sense it in every way possible doing the same. For this method it isn't simply enough to acknowledge the fact of rejuvenation, you have to take it even further by feeling it in every way possible as well.)

Chapter 7

PRAYER

The Background

Prayer allows us to come in contact with our desired level of health. When we pray we expect that what we pray for is real and that it is in our future. When we know for sure that the healing we pray for is possible our prayer is bolstered. And when we doubt that healing is possible we feel less incentive to pray.

When the result of our prayer bolsters our desire to continue to want to pray we say that that prayer is a very effective healing tool. If and when we find such a prayer it behooves us to continue using it to achieve our desired level of health. A prayer like this literally brings us closer to our healing and makes us feel as though, on some level, we've already healed. As we continue to pray and see the results in our healing, we find that our prayed-for healing begins to more and more resemble our present state. And when the healing we pray for becomes the same as our actual healing, then we are said to be able to see, feel and sense our healing in every way possible.

Step 1

See, feel and sense in every way possible that you're coming closer to the achievement of your desired level of health, and only the achievement of your desired level of health.

(Hint: Exclude from this step anything and everything that doesn't happen to match your health goal. Don't ask yourself 'I wonder what my achievement would smell like?' Smell it! Don't ask yourself 'I wonder what my achievement will sound like?' Hear it! Don't ask yourself 'What my achievement will look like?' See it! Don't ask yourself 'What will it feel like?' Touch it! Feel it, sense it, see it, smell it, hear it, because you're not only fully capable and able to achieve it, but you have already achieved it.)

Last Step

Look for the signs that you're coming closer to being healed.

(Hint: Like a long awaited approach of a mountain, the outline of your health goal will become more pronounced as you move closer to your achievement of your optimally desired level of health. That creation is yours to see, to feel and to touch. So, take care and make it look and feel just the way you want it. And when you're satisfied with your creation, come and claim it as your own. It belongs to you.)

Chapter 8

PRAYERS COLLECTION/ PRAYERS RECEPTION

The Background

All around us the universe is teeming with prayers of good will and healing toward others. Many around the world pray for the health of strangers around the world. Do not let this precious fount of prayers energy go to waste during your healing process. The energies of good intentions behind those prayers are very potent.

Consider these prayers as a form of positive higher level vibrations. Also consider that just like everything in this universe, these energies are intelligent and are imbued with consciousness. This means that these prayers can be communicated with and consciously directed by their recipient for their healing. At the very least, these higher vibration thoughts will help you to raise your vibration to where healing ultimately is.

Step 1

See, feel and sense in every way possible that the collective prayers of others around the world are reaching your body and mind, and are busy at work on enabling you to achieve your optimally desired level of health.

(Hint: The energy of prayer is washing over your body and mind, and passing through in abundance as big and as wide as you want. Permit this to happen, and see, feel and sense in every way possible that you're indeed coming to the achievement of your optimally desired level of health.)

Last Step

When you feel up to it, go ahead and join others in their collective prayers for those needing healing. Your gift, in whatever amount you decide to donate it, will be appreciated and be of much use to those in need. That way you will be able to add your jewel to the universal prayer reservoir from our side of the space. And make it freely available to those who desire to achieve their optimally desired level of health.

Chapter 9

COMMUNICATION/CONVERSATION WITH AFFECTED AREA

The Background

The universe is imbued with intelligence and reason behind everything. And nothing is wasted. Everything in the universe has its own level of consciousness and everything has a purpose. Based on this, an illness too has a purpose and is ultimately not a waste. And just like anything else in the universe, it too is imbued with consciousness, and is used by the universe to achieve some purpose.

Having consciousness in the universe means that everything can be communicated with by the use of your consciousness. The physical illness is composed of its own intelligence and consciousness. It communicates with the physical body by sending it health symptoms that may be unpleasant. These health symptoms have a purpose, which is often symbolic and personal to its recipient. Health symptoms act as communication messages that an illness sends to the physical body of the recipient. These messages then can be accepted or ignored.

If the messages are accepted and acted on, then the intelligence behind the message wastes no further time to send them again. This is because nothing in the universe is wasted and everything has a purpose. So, if the purpose of your illness was to give you some message, then once that's done, an illness is free to go toward its own spiritual evolution. If however, you ignore the message that's got your name, then the universe looks for more ways to get you to pay attention. And this means that your physical symptoms might become more exaggerated because you refused to understand the message the first time.

Step 1

Make sure you're really ready to begin communicating with your imbalance or illness. Ask yourself, 'Am I really ready to start the conversation?' Or, 'What is it am I seeking to communicate? Am I ready to receive an answer, or take the time to send anger and hate?'

(Hint: We often insert powerful emotions and feelings into the outputs we send, especially if we feel something really matters. And feelings such as hate, anger, fear and resentment, can cloud, or even incorrectly alter the answers we may receive. Hating an illness or an imbalance, apart from communication, is a very real force that can close the channels. If we want to receive a clear and real answers, the sender must first address these emotions. It's not to say that an imbalance or illness, or its cause must be loved. Only that the focus should shift to openly receiving an answer. Also, remember that freeing deep negative emotions is also a part of ultimately going towards the achievement of your desire level of health.)

Step 2

Ask your particular imbalance, or illness, the following: 'Show and tell me what it is you want to show and tell me'. Keep asking for as long as you need to get the answer. The answer always comes.

(Hint: Feel free to change the suggested wording or improve upon it, or pick the kind of words which you feel best suit your personality. Also, no matter what words you ultimately decide to use, please try and keep your statement as simple and to the point as possible.)

(Hint: If during the course of this initial practice the answer, story or image from the entity you're asking, comes in hazy or goes past your head, then feel free to kindly ask it to show and tell it again in the way you can understand.)

Last Step

Visualize the symbolic representation of the words and questions you seek to ask as much as possible. Especially, as it becomes appropriate to a particular level of communication employed by a particular entity.

(Hint: Be patient with them, just as you would with anyone you've never communicated with before. Just as you need the time to get used to talking to them, they also need the time to get used to your new communication. In time they'll realize you're not kidding around, and will begin to respond. You're, sort of, helping them as much as you're helping yourself, because it's time to move on.)

(Hint: The message is out there for you to receive, and you are receiving it and will receive it whether your mind recognizes it or not. Sometimes, you get the answer on a deeper level, on your soul level, and so you see the achievement of your desired level of health without really recognizing why with your mind. That's ok too. Just remember that the message for you is out there. And whatever that message happens to be, treat it with respect it deserves, or don't ask until you're ready for 'any' answer.)

Chapter 10

LOVING KINDNESS TO THE AFFECTED PART OF THE BODY

The Background

The human body has an amazing way to respond to various thoughts inside the human head. The human body as a whole is a conscious and intelligent organism that sends out and responds to communications. It uses various means to communicate and to receive communication. Additionally, every cell inside the human body also acts in the same way and also sends and receives communication. The cells inside the human body, then, respond in proportion to how they are being treated by a person. They are excellent eavesdroppers and pay attention every time a person thinks or talks about them. Then, they respond to the information they find.

The infected cell, or the cell of an illness are no different in their capacity to absorb information than any other living cell. An illness also has intelligence and consciousness that responds in kind. An illness, therefore, is not 'evil' or 'negative' per say. It's just there to do its 'job'. It appreciates being recognized and being treated with love and kindness just like anything else.

Step 1

Familiarize yourself with what your loving kindness feels like.

(Hint: Take this time to practice loving kindness to your surroundings, some items or people you dearly love. Perhaps it's your house you've designed, your garden, your pet, or your collection.)

Step 2

Now, take that experience of loving kindness and begin to try and shift it toward a part of your body. Find a way in to feel love and kindness toward a part, or parts, of your body and mind.

(Hint: Perhaps you might feel loving kindness toward your appearance, your hair, your eyes; or, maybe your particular personality trait or a skill. Find something about your body and mind that you happen to like. There's got to be something. Look as long and as best as you know how. I guarantee, you do have something you can feel loving kindness toward.)

(Hint: Finding just enough about your body and mind to feel loving kindness toward will open the door for the rest of you. Doing so will give you a foothold to pour your energy of loving kindness on your entire body and mind. Find a reason to feel loving kindness toward a certain part of the body and mind. It doesn't have to be your whole body right away.)

Step 3

Now, expand the feeling of loving kindness toward more and more parts of your body.

Work your way toward including your whole body and mind.

(Hint: Give yourself the permission to gradually experience more and more loving kindness toward your whole body and mind in its entirety.)

Step 4

Expand the same feeling of loving kindness toward those parts of you that are ill and are in need of healing.

Work your way toward allowing the strength, force, power, and tremendous potential of your power of loving kindness to expand toward your particular illness.

(Hint: Cells do hear your thoughts, so it's no use pretending. Enemies are hard to love, but this is the nuts and bolts of this method. Perhaps, doing so might be easier on you if you started with one of the smallest and easily manageable imbalances, or illnesses, of your body and mind. Work your way around the more tolerable edges of your illness first. Take your time doing this, be gentle on yourself, and understand that once you experience loving kindness, you can then go ahead and apply it to anything you wish.)

Last Step

Douse your entire imbalance, or illness, with your energy of loving kindness. Try this right now. Don't wait. You're safe and are achieving your desired level of health anyways. You have nothing to lose.

(Hint: Consider focusing your energy first on one of your

smallest and easily manageable imbalances, or illnesses, and then gradually working your way up toward the larger imbalance, or illness. You have the power of loving kindness to guide you. So, use it to break free from your prejudices and hates.)

Chapter 11

CRYSTAL BALL

The Background

Human beings have a limitless power of creativity. We create all the time. But more often than not our creativity is scattered in many places, or maybe even ignored. Nevertheless, the creativity does exist and can give us great comprehensible results if and when we focus it.

The following method is really about taking this creativity and putting it into a comprehensible form which we can then use to achieve our desired level of health. A crystal ball is just such a shape. For many this shape is very easy to visualize and focus on in the one's mind. It makes for a clear framework in which the power of creativity can expand and be maintained for healing.

Step 1

See yourself surrounded by a clear crystal ball. It's perfect in shape and it's crystal clear. See yourself being fully at one with the ball. It moves where you move and it goes where you go. To the outside its outer wall is as smooth and impenetrable as a diamond. Its inside is of the same consistency, or more malleable if you prefer, and acts like a liquid crystal around you, and merging with you.

Last Step

See if you can change the shape of your crystal ball, or even a tinge. Then, see it expand further beyond your body, perhaps your room, or your house. Or, see its walls vibrate, or revolve it in a particular direction, or give it the outer plasticity you desire.

Chapter 12

CONVERSATION WITH THE HIGHER SELF/ HIGHER CONSCIOUSNESS ON PERCEIVED LESSONS

The Background

Each of us has a Higher Self, aka Higher Consciousness, who directs everything in our lives. It can be thought of as one's own personal God/Goddess to which one can pray and ask for direction. I prefer to view it as one's Spirit who uses one's physical body as its vehicle to accomplish its goals. This includes the experience of what it's like to live here on earth. When the physical body's life is done the Higher Self picks a different body with which to interact and to direct its living.

The Higher self is very aware of what's going on with the human body, or its host, at any time. It has all the answers and is beyond intelligent. The body may be mortal, but not the spirit. All this means that one can communicate with their higher self to find the answers for their particular illness. Often, it's just an experience that the spirit has chosen to have during this life. It knows what illness is all about and what to do in order to find the answers for healing.

First and Last Step

Ask your higher self, higher consciousness, or spirit, or whatever term you're most comfortable with, what lesson your particular imbalance, or illness, is there to teach you. Phrase it in any way you want, and through whatever medium you feel most comfortable with.

(Hint: Keep asking for as long as you need to get the answer. Your Higher Self is a higher you. This means that you have your divine right to communicate with it at your pleasure.)

Chapter 13

IDENTIFYING WITH SELF IN THE FUTURE TENSE/IMBALANCE IS TEMPORARY

The Background

There is no future and no past. There's only NOW. Past is where you're now. Future is where you are now. It's all now. So, if future and past are two major ways in which humans interpret their present, then it is true that there can only be now. And if people simultaneously exits in the future, the present and the now, then that means they must be everywhere at once. And this means that the future must be a part of NOW.

You can change your future by changing your present state. And since the past, the future and the present are all part of your now, then you can 'pre-form' your future and become a part of that future this present moment.

If you know and are certain that you're definitely going to heal your illness in the 'future', while keeping in mind that past and future and present are all interconnected. Then you can certainly have that 'future of health' become your reality NOW.

First and Last Step

See, feel and sense yourself in every way possible as having already achieved your desired level of health. Connect with that future as much as possible.

(Hint: Work your way up by practicing this method on one of your smallest imbalances, or illness. And then, once you get better at it, move on to the imbalance which would require more concentration and focus. It's ok to first acquire some confidence in your knowledge about the relative perception of time.)

(Hint: Every time something unpleasant happens, practice the same technique. And don't just believe that your future is certain. Embrace it, <u>feel it in every way possible</u> as though it has already come. And KNOW that it is so. The more you know this, the more natural it will be for you to feel yourself in the future, or the 'now' of your own making.)

Chapter 14

HEALING VISUALIZATION

The Background

What you see is what you get. We visualize things in our minds all the time. And we do it so naturally that often we even forget the distinction between what we consider to be 'real' and that which we had merely expected to see. We look for things we want to see. We readily look for things which reinforce our conclusions and avert our eyes from things that contradict what we want to see.

Visualization works because we see things before they happen to us, or else become blind to those things which we have no comprehension of. And when we have no concept of something then we will literally be blind to it even if it's brought right before our eyes. On the other hand, if we are familiar with something, then we will instantly recognize it even if it shows up in our peripheral vision.

At a deeper sense, visualization aids us in 'creating' that which we want to see. Visualization with our mind is how we create things. All this makes visualization an extremely potent tool which we can use to clearly define our health goals, and also to give our creativity a framework in which it can then begin to operate and keep focused. Visualization skill also means that if we visualize something we really don't want to see, then that too will be created into our perceived sense of reality.

First and Last Step

Whatever your particular imbalance, or illness, happens to be, simply visualize it in every way you can being healed.

(Hint: Work your way up in your visualization skills by beginning to apply this method to simpler imbalances first, where visualizing may be much easier. Then progressively move toward your bigger imbalances. Of course, that's just a suggestion, because visualization happens in our mind all the time. And there's really no telling what you can see.)

(Hint: Using your imagination is not forbidden. So, go ahead and feel free to make the kind of imaginary images of healing that best make sense to you. If it helps you, consider coming up with a storyline which illustrates healing.)

Chapter 15

COSMIC RAIN SHOWER OF LIGHT VISUALIZATION

The Background

The universe is full of healing energy. This energy is conscious and intelligent. This energy is free for the taking. And it responds to intelligent and conscious interaction from us, just like any other conscious and intelligent matter in the universe.

In a simple sense, this healing energy is there for us to use. And it is also the energy that nourishes and sustains us throughout our lives. We need this energy in order to grow and in order to heal. And since it has intelligence and consciousness it is in its nature to communicate and to be directed toward our healing. By consciously interacting with this energy we can better direct it toward those areas of the body which need healing.

First and Last Step

Take this moment to see yourself being washed over and through by the cosmic rain shower of light. See it washing over your body in an abundant stream. See it cleansing your entire body and filling in the voids which you feel need to be filled. See it washing over your particular imbalance, or illness, cell by cell, and even inside each cell. Keep seeing it as long as you desire to do so.

Chapter 16

WHITE LIGHT OF PROTECTION AND CLEANSING

The Background

When we think of white light we often picture purity and clarity. These and many like synonyms are no coincidence why we all have these nearly identical associations with the image of 'white light'. This is because these associations with certain colors are prewired into us.

For example, why do doctors and priests around the world wear white robes? Or, why is the color of healing and medical cures represented with white? White is a very sterile color which naturally lends itself to being stained, but also, in its purest form, it is the best background color against which any discoloration or blemish is readily perceived. All colors serve their purpose and are very important. But sometimes it's simply our gut feeling, our intuition if you will, which tells us what color seems more appropriate for a particular function. Beyond all this is the fact that colors are symbolic representations of the Spiritual and cosmic plane of existence. And the color white just happens to be best suited to the function of spotting and removing of blemishes. Illnesses can be viewed as the sort of 'blemishes' on the body, and point the way to the imbalance.

The added function of colors is that they can be easily visualized and help bring in a certain frame of mind. White light is just such a color. Thinking on it, or better yet visualizing it, is just another way which gives us a simple and easy target to raise our physical vibration to the energetic vibration of the color white. When our mind is at the vibration of the white light, the vibration of the white light does what it is meant to do. It heals and purifies.

Step 1

Say the following two sayings in your mind, 'Thank you, divine spirit, for surrounding me with your white light of protection', and 'Thank you, divine spirit, for cleansing me with your white light of cleansing'.

(Hint: Another variation of this can also go like this, 'Thank you, divine spirit, for cleansing me with your white light of complete bodily cleansing', or 'Thank you, divine spirit, for cleansing me with your white light of complete mental cleansing'.)

(Hint: Keep in mind that these sayings are just suggestions, so feel free to come up with your own variations on the wording you like.)

Last Step

As you say the sayings above in your mind, or those sayings which respond better to your personality, also consider trying to see in your mind what those sayings describe as best as you can.

(Hint: Thinking and seeing something gives you more senses with which to tune in to, and create your target vibration rate.)

Chapter 17

RAINBOW LIGHT OF CLEANSING AND COMPLETE HEALING

The Background

Each primary color, or a blend of colors, all around you is there by no accident. Each color clearly denotes a particular use in nature for which it is designed. Each color has its own particular vibration. And this makes every color appropriate and necessary.

Just as the universe and the earth nature around us has colors, so are the colors of various parts of our body clearly designated. In a simplified way, this is because our body is a miniature version of the universe. The universe has many colors which to us form into an orderly rainbow that has all of the primary colors and many colors in between. Each of the colors of the rainbow has its own energetic vibration that is in tune with a particular color of each part of the human body. And each part of the human body is denoted by its own optimal vibration.

And just like in the larger universe, in the body the particular colors suggest a particular vibration at which each part of the body must vibrate in order to perform at its optimal function. The discoloration or fading of these colors are an important indication of how well the body part is performing. When each part of the body vibrates at its own rate they are said to display their own unique function. Like a well-tuned symphony, these separate vibrations all come together to form what we refer to as the human body.

The added function of colors is that they can be easily visualized and help bring in a certain frame of mind. Thinking of all of the colors at once, or better yet visualizing them as a type of rainbow, is just another way which gives us a simple and easy target to raise our whole physical vibration at once. When our mind is at the vibration of all the colors, the vibration of all the colors at once does what it is designed to do. It tunes each part of the physical body with energetic vibration of their appropriate color. This in turn realigns the whole body into its desired blend of vibrations and brings all of the colors to their optimal freshness.

Step 1

Say the following two sayings in your mind, 'Thank you, divine spirit, for cleansing me with your rainbow light of cleansing', and 'Thank you, divine spirit, for cleansing me with your rainbow light of complete bodily healing'.

(Hint: These sayings are just suggestions, so feel free to come up with your own variations on the wording you like.)

Last Step

As you say the sayings above in your mind, or those sayings which respond better to your personality, also consider trying to see in your mind what those sayings describe as best as you can.

(Hint: Consider visualizing an abundant assortment of colorful rainbow lights, as vibrant as you want them to be. Likewise, if you feel a need for a particular color, then have that assortment of lights predominate with a particular color. For example, if you need to help your heart or relax your mind, then let those round blotches, dots or specks of light, or whatever visual you're most comfortable with, be interspersed with more shades of green.)

Chapter 18

VORTEX ENERGY HEALING

The Background

The material world we live in is not the whole picture of how the universe really works. In simple terms, everything has its counterpart in order to function and remain alive. Male/Female, left/right, positive/negative are just some of the most obvious examples. And their number is really as infinite as the universe, because everything has to have its opposite to stay alive. To complicate things a bit more let's say that in addition to its material counterpart, every material thing in this universe also has its spiritual counterpart. In general this counterpart is known as the spiritual world, or what some call heaven. The counterpart of our material world is the spiritual world.

The Spiritual World may very well function independent of the material world. However, the material world would not be possible without its spiritual counterpart. This is because everything originated in the spiritual world, and this even includes the material world. The degree of how 'material' things are in this universe shows in how close a given thing is to its spiritual counterpart. Or, how close in consciousness (vibration) something is to the spiritual world.

The material world communicates with the spiritual world. And the spiritual world is really in charge of how all of the things in the material world get manifested. In order for this creative process to work smoothly, the spiritual world needs a directing assistant (aka its counterpart) in the material world. This type of creation process is alive and well, and it happens nonstop. The material world is created through certain portals that exist everywhere there's a material thing. The spiritual world uses these portals (aka spirals or vortexes) to communicate with the material world, and to adjust it as needed. These vortex gateways are like doors that are used to exchange and pass information to create or de-create a matter.

These portals are intelligent in themselves and are guided by the creative spiritual beings to exchange and to receive new information. When healing happens, these portals are used like invisible 'umbilical' chords to send the physical body the information it needs to get well. An intelligent being, like human, is possessed of conscience and spirituality. This enables a person to consciously communicate with the spiritual world through the portals, and to thus better assist themselves in their healing process. This communication happens all the time, but its effect can be very amplified when the being on the earth side is especially conscious of the exchange. When two consciousnesses meet together great healing happens.

Step 1

Go ahead and simply visualize a clockwise spiral moving away from your physical body and pointing away from it to form a pointed cone.

(Hint: This is the <u>sending</u> of material energy, or the information about an illness.)

(Hint: Practice doing this a couple of times to get the hang of it.)

Step 2

Now, holding the same clockwise spiral in your mind, place it over the particular area of your body and mind, which you feel is in need of the <u>removal</u> of your particular imbalance, or illness.

(Hint: If you can't place your illness, place the vortex over your entire body.)

Step 3

Now, change your visual image by visualizing a counterclockwise spiral moving toward your physical body, or toward its particular part. Practice doing this a couple of times to get the hang of it.

(Hint: This is the <u>receiving</u> of spiritual energy, or the healing information.)

(Hint: Instead of narrowing away from your physical body, this spiral widens toward its base where it touches your physical body. Its pointed, or narrowing side, however, still points away from your body.)

Last Step

Now, holding the same counterclockwise spiral in your mind, place it over a particular area of your body, where the healing is needed. So, perhaps, you injured something and the injury is clean, but you still feel you need rapid boost in mending it. Likewise, feel free to place this spiral over your entire body for overall balance.

Chapter 19

DIVINE HAND VISUALIZATION

The Background

This method can work well for those who are just beginning to work on their healing visualization skills. It's an easy way to start because visualizing a human hand is very easy to do. We can even use our own hands as a model.

Also, many can readily understand the association between the comfort of hands and healing. Hands are what give and nurture us when we are young. And they are important healing tools when it comes to any kind of energy work. In fact, many types of miraculous healings are still done through hands. Some say that the reason this is so is because the center of human hands has an important chakra point that acts like a wire to transmit healing energy.

First and Last Step

See your body and mind, or a particular part of your body and mind, being gently touched and surrounded by the divine hand. If it helps you, go ahead and feel free to see an actual human-like hand being placed over your body and mind, that's all fine. Or, feel free to give it a particular tinge, or keep it colorless and translucent if that suites you. Keep seeing that energy as long as you need, comforting you and watching over you.

Chapter 20

FORGIVING

The Background

No healing is possible without truly forgiving. In the simplest terms, to forgive means to give-before. Another way to think of it is as giving away or letting go of something. Because when you truly forgive or let go of something, then you shouldn't be bothered by it again. And forgiveness of others begins with the forgiveness of self.

Healing is very much about how much we are willing to forgive ourselves. Having an illness is an imbalance manifested, and is not the most optimal physical state. Neither is it the 'normal' state of the body. An illness indicates that something's out of whack, and indicates an imbalance. An illness is also what a person does to themselves. And often, it indicates that a person is not doing to themselves what they need to do. In that sense, illness is a kind of self-hurt. When we forgive ourselves, truly forgive ourselves, then our self-hurting illness will outlive its usefulness. Then it will also be easier to forgive other beings, and let go of the self-poisoning thoughts in our lives.

Step 1

Take this moment to glance over your entire life, as far back as you can. Try to remember the situations, things, or people that you may have perceived wronged you, attacked you or caused you to feel upset.

(Hint: Begin with the simplest one you can understand. Perhaps, it was an unpleasant dialogue you might have had with someone when you were younger and you feel you would have answered more aggressively to feel better now. Try to understand as best you can what it was that caused you to perceive that you were wronged, attacked, or felt upset.)

Last Step

Once you find a particular situation, thing or a person worthy of your forgiveness, then try to see if you can intentionally forgive those circumstances, that event, that thing or that person, or persons. If you feel you can forgive, then try your best to forgive in your mind and consciously acknowledge that you've done so. Then, once you're ready to review another event, go ahead and do so again, again, again. Understand then forgive, understand then forgive, understand then forgive.

(Hint: Forgiveness is a gradual process, and understanding takes effort. So be easy on yourself now so you won't have to feel you'll need to forgive yourself later. But if you have to, be generous and forgive yourself. Only you can forgive yourself.)

Chapter 21

REGRETLESSNESS

The Background

How can you feel better about yourself and also be held by oppressive and bitter thoughts? Even if you do that, won't you still have some regrets still left in your life?

The regrets, however small, have a way of haunting us and coming to bite at our self-assuredness. This is because all regrets have a thought residue that is not conducive to our optimal level of health. Oftentimes, these thoughts are so strong that they can become an actual illness. And in that case, letting go of what caused those feelings in the first place becomes of utmost importance to regain our balanced health.

First and Last Step

Look over your life, beginning with the simplest possible regret. Then see if you can let go of that regret, or readily resolve the situation that caused it, or is causing it. Once you get good at this, then go ahead and see if you can find a way to let go of your larger regrets. The overall goal is to have as few regrets in your life as possible

(Hint: Letting go of regrets does not mean that you have to deny such things as an abusive relationship, or the career which degrades the majesty of who you are, or tolerate a toxic environment, etc. It doesn't, but you can still go ahead and change those things without having to have your regrets drag you down.)

Chapter 22

THE UNIVERSAL DECLARATION: I CHOOSE TO BE IN BALANCE

The Background

Every human is a conscious and spiritual being, endowed with a free will. This free will is given to us, because we are made in the image of the spirit that created us. This spirit has a free will, and this means that we too have a free will to do or not to do as we see fit.

In a broader sense, our individual free will is a very powerful creative force which the material universe obeys. What we 'will' to create becomes manifested. We literally will into existence the things we see around us. On the other hand, we must also live with the consequences of the actions that our free will has generated.

The good thing is that we don't have to continue with the life we created as is without end. We can recreate it and again use our free will to create what we want to happen. So, if we recall that we are the ones who have willed into the existence "the same old" situation of illness in our lives, and are tired of it. Then we likewise have the sovereign willpower to un-will it and make something else.

First and Last Step

Simply say to yourself something like this, 'I choose to be in balance'.

(Hint: Feel free to come up with your own best wording. When you come up with your alternative phrase try to do your best to have it sum up exactly what it is you want. For example, if it's to achieve your optimally desired level of health from your illness, then go ahead and choose the kind of statement which gets straight to the point of what it is you want, and only what you want. Keep it as positive as you can and have that statement say only what you want to achieve, and at the exclusion of anything and everything that doesn't happen to match only your optimally desired healing.)

Chapter 23

BELIEVING

The Background

The healing version of reality competes with other 'realities' for our attention. Among them is an illness version of reality. When we are ill we are convinced by our health symptoms. And when we are healing we are convinced by the waning of the symptoms. It's like a tug of war, and ultimately one vision of reality prevails. What we see we believe – What we believe we see. The more convinced we are that something is going on the more likely we are to accept that version of reality. When we are convinced we're ill it becomes our reality. And, when we're convinced we are healing it becomes our reality.

In basic terms, our beliefs are an example of very complex thoughts (aka thought forms). These complex thought forms are much more influential than the average run of the mill thoughts in that they determine how our mind will process later thoughts or ideas. Our frame of mind then is the place where we can receive and process various thoughts and ideas.

Every thought form has its own particular vibration. And these thoughts come together based on their similar vibrations. When enough of these thoughts come together they form into complex version of themselves. In this way the beliefs are an example of these complex thought forms.

Whether we accept or reject a particular thought form depends very much on whether or not that thought form's vibration matches with the overall vibration of our frame of mind. Conversely, the overall vibration of our frame of mind is made up of many like thoughts. The presence of these thought forms is what nourishes and sustains the continued function of our frame of mind. Like attracts like, and so when our frame of mind is made of beliefs (aka complex thought forms) that have a strong vibration, these in turn determine how our mind will process incoming thoughts and ideas. When the vibration of our thoughts and our frame of mind reaches the same level, then the overall vibration for the rest of our physical bodies is created. So that ultimately, our thoughts, minds and bodies operate at the same vibration. When they do, they then set the level of how we perceive our physical reality. And at what vibration that reality happens to operate.

When, for example, a person believes they are ill and that they can't heal, they've set up how they choose to view their reality. It begins with the thoughts they choose to accept. If they accept enough of the negative thoughts of lower vibration, such as illness, these thoughts form together into beliefs (aka more complex thought forms) that they are ill. The vibration of these thought forms then impacts the overall vibration of their frame of mind, and how it filters incoming ideas. And so, if the vibration is negative, then this means that the overall vibration of their frame of mind is lowered. Then, when the vibration of their thoughts and their frame of mind reaches the same negative level, this sets up the vibration for the rest of their body. Like attracts like, and a physical body that operates at this negative vibration will begin to get ill. When this thought cycle is completed the reality that that person is ill is created. And it will continue to operate at that lower vibration until they choose to switch their vibration.

Our particular reality is based on our choice. And we can choose how we want to form our beliefs (aka complex thought forms) based on which thoughts we choose to accept and which to reject. When we choose to raise the vibration of our reality, then that creates a framework to form our beliefs out of similar thoughts of higher vibration. So that by raising the vibration of our beliefs with the thoughts of healing and rejuvenation, the vibration of our frame of mind is then raised to that level as well. With the vibration of our beliefs and frame of mind operating at the same higher level, this will then set the tone for the higher vibration for the rest of our bodies. So that when the vibration of our beliefs, our frame of mind and our bodies vibrate at the same higher level, the higher vibration of our reality will be created. On the other hand, if we choose to form our beliefs only with the thoughts of illness, then it will be reflected in our chosen frame of mind, which will then influence how our bodies will end up sensing the reality.

Step 1

Define your ultimate healing goal by coming up with a statement which would suggest to you that you have already healed. For example, it might be a simple statement like 'I am healed from such and such'.

(Hint: Try and keep your statement simple by limiting your statement to an easily spoken one-liner. It will make it easier to focus on.)

(Hint: You're saying your statement to yourself in order to get a clear idea of what your healing is going to be.)

Step 2

Select the first sign that will make you believe that you're actually beginning to see the improvement in your overall condition.

(Hint: The first sign of your improvement doesn't have to be the kind that would be necessarily recognized or agreed upon by any other person except you. The particular size of the sign is not as important as its ability to readily demonstrate to you that you are achieving your desired level of health. All it has to do is be just sufficient enough of a proof to have <u>you</u> begin to believe that you are actually healing.)

(Hint: Your sign may be as simple as seeing your emotional state adjust for the better, or it may be the reduction in pain, irritation or anything like that. Simpler sign is better here, because it will give you more chances of being demonstrated.)

Step 3

Find a confirmation, no matter how small, that your predetermined sign has materialized.

(Hint: You're working to help yourself believe that you can heal. That's the team you're working for. That's the reality you've chosen to see.)

(Hint: Be flexible and keep readjusting your sign. Come up with a new sign and even reduce the size of your chosen sign. Do whatever it takes for you to see it become real. Break those little signs so far down into their smaller parts, or goals, or steps, or journeys, that your belief in yourself and your ability to achieve them becomes so unshakable that all you'll have left to do is just achieve them.)

(Hint: Be on the alert for the possibility that the improvement in your physical condition may be demonstrated by any number of signs. Some of them you may not have thought of before.)

Step 4

Now go ahead and say without the least shadow of a doubt, 'I am healing'. Or, find your own convincing enough statement which will be utterly impossible for you to deny. Just find a statement you can't deny even if you tried.

(Hint: If your sign has come true, sure you can say it. If you need more evidence, then come up with more signs to be fulfilled. But believing that you can heal is your ultimate goal. Your doubts are beliefs too, and you've spent a long time reinforcing them. That's why they seem 'real'. So respect them and understand they may not change overnight.)

(Hint: Look for permissive present tense phrases. These phrases might sound like 'I am rebalancing', or 'My health is improving', etc.)

(Hint: If your sign has come true, acknowledge it with the kind of statement that recognizes your achievement of shifting to the alternative belief. Treat your proof with the respect it deserves. And nourish and protect your sprouting belief. Healing often begins with just a small step.)

Last Step

Look for other small proofs to reinforce your personal belief in yourself and your ability to begin to achieve your desired level of health.

(Hint: No matter how grandiose the ultimate healing may be, it's always made up of smaller improvements.)

(Hint: If it helps, think of it as not trying to convince yourself that you're healed, or even to force yourself to believe that your optimally desired level of health is even possible. No, here you're just seeking out sufficient enough demonstrations of your improvement in order for you to continue to believe what you believe anyways. That you are healing.)

Chapter 24

STAYING POSITIVE

The Background

When you're motivated and inspired about something it sure is easy to stay positive. But what is healing other than a positive thing? The very notion of healing inspires us to look for cures and go the sometimes long and arduous journey to achieve our desired level of health. This is what true healing does, it motivates and inspires. And healing is synonymous with positivity.

During an illness however, it's very difficult to stay positive. It's hard to get motivated and inspired to do something when you haven't found the cure. And when everything you've tried just doesn't seem to work. The added pressure to staying positive also happens when our mental and physical energy are drained by an illness. And we just don't want to do anything.

And yet, at the first sign that we're healing, the positivity snaps up again. And we instantly have a surge of motivation and inspiration. Conversely, with illness the positivity declines. This is because staying positive is a frame of mind. And any frame of mind attracts to itself the like things. For example, a positive frame of mind attracts positive qualities to itself. Conversely, a negative frame of mind attracts negative qualities while repelling the positive.

So, if it's healing you want then you must get yourself into the mental state that will attract the healing you want. Give yourselves more and more reasons to feel positive to not only achieve your healing, but also to go on achieving your healing. Find the reasons that motivate and inspire you to continue healing. Look for and find any clues that you're healing. You have to continue to stay positive in order to get to the vibration you want.

Step 1

Name your illness. Come up with the most accurate name possible to describe your illness.

(Hint: Here you're trying to get a better idea of what's going on with you.)

Step 2

Now focus on coming up with the best goal statement to describe what healing you want to achieve. Describe only what healing you want to achieve and at the exclusion of anything that doesn't match that goal.

(Hint: The easiest way to do this is to come up with the complete opposite of the negative description of your illness. For example, if you're ill or unhealthy, or have a particular imbalance, then here you can go ahead and try to come up with the completely opposite statement. For example, the opposite of ill would be healthy, the opposite of aging would be rejuvenated, and the opposite of problem would be solution.)

(Hint: Exclude from your goal statements No's, Not's and Less's. For example, don't even waste your time saying to yourself statements like, 'I'm not ill', 'I'm feeling less and less ill', or 'I'm not aging', or 'My problem is going away'. This would just be wasting your energy and time on trying to deny what you already know is obvious. Instead, really try and look for a clever way to paraphrase, switch, or convert the negative undesired condition into your desired goal to find healing. This way you'll have something positive to look forward to achieving, something that will motivate and inspire you to achieve it.)

Last Step

Find more positive reasons to feel motivated and inspired about achieving your healing. Give yourself more and more reasons to feel positive, motivated and inspired about achieving your healing. These reasons may include the first tiny proofs that you're healing.

(Hint: Do not confuse staying positive with using your negative illness symptoms to frighten yourself into being 'positively motivated and inspired' to get healthy. Staying positive is about putting your focus on your ultimate health goal.)

Chapter 25

MAKING YOUR INTENT

The Background

Having an intention to achieve healing is an indispensable tool that enables us to focus and concentrate on what it is exactly we want to achieve. And without a focus and concentration it is impossible to achieve anything. The greater our intent on something, the more likely we will achieve something. That's because greater intention brings greater focus and concentration. And greater focus and concentration on that which we want to achieve ensures that more of our energy is brought to bear toward that vision of reality which we want to create.

When someone really intends to get well they bring their focus and concentration on being healed. Health is a balanced frame of mind. And so when we focus and concentrate on achieving more balance we automatically raise our vibration to match that level. The more we intend something, the more real it becomes and the more time we spend there. When we spend more and more time in a healthy frame of mind, the more it becomes natural to us. And the more we want to be there without taking it for granted. Like attracts like, so, the more time we spend there the closer our vibration gets to that level. When our vibration matches with the vibration of our intent, it becomes that thing.

Step 1

Clear your mind from any intrusion whatsoever, and try to get as relaxed and as calm as possible by freeing your mind from anything else that might come to distract your fullest attention on what you're about to do.

Step 2

Come up with words and description which might best define your desired health goal.

(Hint: Come up something that would begin to define and clarify your desired goal.)

Step 3

<u>See</u>, <u>feel</u> and <u>sense in every way possible</u> that you are already achieving you desired goal. Clearly visualize or clearly sense what your ultimate goal is actually going to be.

(Hint: Your ultimate health goal doesn't even necessarily have to be summed up by a perfect sounding statement to really bring the intention home. Perhaps, it's just seeing your skin clear from the blemish symptoms of some skin irritation. Whatever it is, be as specific as you possibly can.)

(Hint: Feelings, visions and sensations help crystallize what it is you actually want to achieve. They can give you just the focus and concentration you need in order to go about achieving it.)

Step 4

Bring as much of your focus and concentration on only your ultimately desired health goal as if it actually already happened. Immerse yourself in that feeling and become familiar with it.

(Hint: Stay in the target vibration you want.)

Last Step

Come up with a statement that best defines your desired goal as if you're achieving it or have already achieved it. For example, you might think to yourself, 'I am healing', or 'I am beginning to heal'.

(Hint: Include in your definition of your desired goal only that which you actually want to achieve. So, saying 'I will', or 'I'm going to', brings your attention back toward your illness or situation which you're trying to overcome in the first place.)

Chapter 26

BEING CREATIVE

The Background

Brick by brick, pen stroke by pen stoke, hour by hour, we create. With every note we create that music which stirs and inspires the very heart of humanity. As you walk on a sandy tropical beach you're actually witnessing the very definition of creativity. Sand grain by sand grain, water drop by water drop, leaf by leaf, our experience is made wonderful and precious. How about the stars? They too are made up of the infinity of other like particles which repeatedly combined to form into a one cohesive whole of creation, the picture of our lives we enjoy.

Healing is made up of a compellation of many achievements. You can think of those achievements as the smaller version of the ultimate healing itself. Each of those smaller healings is necessary to bring the whole picture together, and none can be excluded. When you achieve even a smaller healing you place yourself on the way to completing your journey to your ultimate health destination.

Healing is a creative process. It's like painting. To paint you need a brush, a canvas, and paints, etc. That can be thought of as your physical body and all the tools you have at your disposal. Then, you prepare your canvas by making your sketch. You might readjust your sketch and draw what you like, because ultimately it's going to be covered by paint. Then, once you've got your rough sketch you begin to lay paint. As you get closer to your finished product you find more clarity about what it is you ultimately looked for. This means that your painting might end up looking differently from what you've originally sketched. And you might be surprised how well it turns out.

The achievement of your desired level of health is likewise a creative process. First, you sketch out the rough idea of what your healing will look like on your canvas of the mind. Then, once that becomes clear enough, you begin to lay on paint by creating the feeling and thoughts for your painting. With every new touch of creativity your painting more and more resembles your final goal. A while later your desired level of health is achieved.

Step 1

Come up with the kind of statement that would best describe the achievement of your desired healing.

(Hint: For example, a statement like, 'I want to achieve healing', although sounds positive, is also a little bit passive and is not really using the fullest potential of the power of creativity to its limitless potential. Likewise, a statement like 'I am healing', is again a bit passive, or as creative as it can possibly be. Pour your creativity into it and you'll see the result.)

(Hint: Do not include in your statement any inkling of anything that might actually in any way oppose your ultimately desired goal. A statement like, 'My sickness is being cured', or 'I'm successfully overcoming my illness', and so on, needlessly takes away your power of creativity and splits it, so to speak, between your desired goal and your imbalance. Be creative, be imaginative and come up with just the statement you feel will be enough for you to really want to create. Go all the way. The power of creativity is at your command. So, exploit it to its fullest extent possible in creating for you your ultimately desired level of health.)

(Hint: A statement to go for might sound something like, 'I am healing more and more', or 'Every day in every way I'm healing more and more and more', or 'My body and mind are healing by leaps and bounds more and more and more each and every day'. See how these statements make you feel, because they are so expanding. In other words, instead of limiting your power of creativity they give it space to roam free, and do what the power of creativity does best when it's set free.)

(Hint: Use words, like 'More', 'Better', 'Every day', 'Leaps and bounds' and so on in the present tense. For example, 'I will be healed by leaps and bounds more and more and more', still diverts some of your power of creativity from your desired goal by pointing to the uncertainty of your situation, not to mention your current condition that has really nothing to do with you ultimately desired goal. Put all your power of creativity on just your ultimately desired goal. 'I'm healing', or 'My body and mind are healing', dot, dot, dot and then the rest is a good example to follow.)

Last Step

Give your power of creativity the direction and space in which it can begin to operate and do its thing. <u>See</u>, <u>feel</u> and <u>sense in every way possible</u> what healing you want to take place. Be creative. Make the achievement of that goal seem as real to you as it can possibly get. Make it come alive. By doing so you come closer to your achievement.

(Hint: Healing depends very much on how you repeatedly create, or achieve all of the other steps which make up that final achievement. It may be that those steps may involve consultation with a medical practitioner, or it may be in the form of taking some supplements, or going through some treatments, or learning specific exercises. Whatever those may be, know that the successful creation of each and every one of them, no matter how small, is ultimately the process of creation of your entire ultimately desired goal.)

(Hint: The achievement of any desired goal is made up of the repeated achievement of all of the other goals which are all a part of your entire and final creation. And so, with this in mind, continue to call on the power of creativity in the achievement of those in-between goals, just as surely as you would in achieving your ultimately desired goal. Don't put the power of creativity to rest simply because you might feel down or upset. Use it to achieve the small as well as your big goals.)

(Hint: Just because the achievement of those smaller goals, or steps on your way to your final achievement of your desired level of health seems easy, do not sneer at them or ridicule them in any way. And understand that without the achievement of those steps, your entire creation would not exist. Address the achievement of all the smaller goals which make up your larger goals. Give them all the necessary degree of respect and attention that they deserve by supplying them with your maximum possible power of creativity to help bring them into being.)

Chapter 27

THE LAST THOUGHT OF THE DAY

The Background

Be kind to yourself. You might have just had a tough day. For some that may make them feel that they haven't come any closer to their achievement of their desired level of health. If that's the case, then remember, that such a belief is a lie, and it doesn't have to be your truth. You are coming closer to your achievement. Of that I'm certain. You're coming closer to your achievement each and every day! Every time you do something, anything, you're coming closer to your achievement. Remember this!

Whatever your day has brought, or whether you're just new to this method, you will get better and better at shifting your thoughts, senses, visions, feelings, or anything else for that matter, on only the achievement of your desired level of health. And at the exclusion of anything and everything that doesn't happen to match only that goal. As you do so, understand that you can take as long a time as you need to get used to this method. Because, just changing your thinking, of that you can be certain, brings you closer to your achievement. It's that easy. Really!

Step 1

Learn to regard your bedding process as a very sacred and important time, which impacts not only the rest of your night, but also the overall healing you will accomplish the next day. So, take this step to prepare yourself and your mind for when you're going to go to bed.

(Hint: How you are going to end your day on a positive note? Don't procrastinate, but begin to think about some of the things which you expect will come to mind when you're back in bed. Contemplate some of the changes you'll make in your overall bedding routine.)

Step 2

Now, try to think to yourself about what it is exactly you might say to yourself to make you feel better and make you feel relaxed and reassured that you're indeed achieving your desired level of health. Make it into a statement or a series of statements that will help put your mind at ease that you're indeed healing.

(Hint: Are you one of those people who always feel that something always comes up unexpected right before you relax? If you know you're prone to this sort of thing, or that there's an event that might trigger those thoughts, then do not let the nightmare spiral out of control. Sit down, and just give yourself the permission to analyze all of the things that can possibly detract you from healing. But do so with a mind that you're going to make an honest effort to reassure yourself that you're in fact alright.)

Last Step

As you're about to have your last thoughts of the day, guide your mind to gently drift toward the healing you want to achieve.

(Hint: Practice what you've prepared. And, if necessary, take mental notes to see how well you're doing and where you might still improve.)

(Hint: If you put your mind to it you will quickly get in the habit of only focusing on the achievement of your desired level of health as your last thought of the day. If you have, you will see, sense, and feel in every way possible that you're coming to the achievement of your desired level of health. Keep it up!)

79

ADDITIONAL NOTES FOR EACH METHOD

1. *The first thought of the day*

Every time we awake is symbolic of being born. We encounter a brand new day and how we decide to begin that day is going to determine the overall character of the rest of the day. The awakening is also analogous to reincarnation experience. When a person wakes up it's as though they had just reincarnated again. Everything they have on a physical and mental level at that time is drawn from the experiences of the previous days.

For many, waking up is a process which they have come to regret because of their illness. And in this way, the process of waking up has come to serve as a reminder of what's wrong with their life. They wake up and see themselves in the same room and in the same day as before, and feel that nothing changed much. The body that houses their soul remains unchanged. So, life's not worth living. They feel that striving to improve their life is useless because they're going to end up in the same place as before. Or, maybe worse.

When a person wakes up with the same illness day and day out, they grow frustrated with themselves. They come to believe that since they've always been ill and since they've never recovered, the healing is not going to occur. Except that they don't realize that since they created their illness and how they feel about it, they also have the ability to un-create it. They just have to know how.

The good news is that healing is possible. If someone wants to see their healing take place, they have to try and snap out of the same old, same old pattern. Unfortunately, 'snapping out' is not so easy if that's all a person is used to. A person has grown accustomed to their ways of thinking and doing things. They've become an expert at being ill and forgot what it's like to feel healed. And they really don't want to change anything because they are afraid of worse things that could happen.

So, perhaps, it's much easier to wake up and begin cursing at the world and the illness. This way they can 'let their frustration out'. But in taking this easy route, a person will not be able to heal. This is because healing is about change. And the change is what needs to occur in order to shift their attention and focus from illness and onto the positive thoughts of healing. Reinforcing how badly they feel about their illness will not allow their mind to find a healing focus.

One of the first things that anyone can start doing on their way to recovery is to reexamine how their day starts. If, for example, their day causes them an illness or does not help them to heal, then maybe the cure rests in how they begin their normal day.

If someone is in earnest, then it really won't take them too long to realize that chances are, they usually begin their day in an unpleasant way. This realization is an important one, because it will give them a strong insight that it's actually their thinking that is to blame for them feeling ill.

The truth is that our thoughts ultimately instruct our bodies how to behave. If, for example, we curse ourselves and our illness when we wake up, we set ourselves up in the wrong thought vibration. And if we do this enough time, these thoughts will begin to harden and materialize into illnesses. In this way we will fight against the natural current of our thoughts and have no way of transcending over our condition.

Mind is a powerful thing when it comes to creating an illness. But it can also be used to create the healing. The difference being is that one person uses their mind to create an illness, while another person uses the same mind to take responsibility for their thoughts in order to heal. This is an important skill that can't be ignored when it comes to healing.

So, instead of taking their first minutes of the morning for granted, a person who desires healing, can use this time of day to skillfully instruct their body to heal. With thoughts like that they will begin to notice the difference in how the rest of their day goes and they will find that they'll be more receptive to healing. As they continue down this path and change their morning routine into a positive frame of mind, it will gradually become a habit. Their thoughts will grow more and more positive, which will in turn raise the vibration of their frame of mind. Then, with their frame of mind operating at a higher vibration, their body will be instructed to likewise operate at a raised vibration. Like attracts like. And so they will have more reasons to feel positive. Then, when they feel positive, they will naturally attract the positive healing vibration to take place. The overall vibration of their physical body will match the overall vibration of healing and they will get well.

2. *Letting go of anger*

If you're bothered by angry thoughts, then rest assured that those thoughts will eventually take a toll on your body.

Overall, anger in our society is usually very rampant and pernicious. In a way it can be thought of as a virus that is widespread. In our society where feelings of anger are often celebrated in the media there is always more than plenty to go around. This means that a person who is unaware of the power of the mind will carelessly expose their frame of mind to the viral thoughts. When someone is exposed to anger and is unaware of what's going on, the natural defenses of their frame of mind wear out. This gradually makes their physical body more vulnerable to the lower vibration anger thoughts. Sometimes, all it takes is just being around chronically angry people for an otherwise healthy person to become ill. They may not even know what caused an illness in the first place.

In reexamining a lot of relationships and how someone has gotten ill, chances are that many will find that at the time, or preceding their illness, they were exposed to an angry atmosphere. Perhaps it was their family members or their work environment. Over time these things take their toll.

Once the thoughts of anger enter your environment, they'll have more chances of entering your mind. Then, once in your mind, an angry thought will have more chances of lowering the overall vibration of your frame of mind. The lowered vibration of the frame of mind will in turn break the health defenses of your body by instructing it to operate at a lower negative vibration. This lowered physical vibration will match the lower vibration of illness and manifest this lowered physical vibrations as an experience of physical illness. This is a very subtle process.

We all have to be careful. And we have become aware when we're in an angry environment. We must not take our natural physical defenses for granted and leave our frames of mind carelessly exposed. After we immerse ourselves enough time in a lowered negative vibration, our minds will change. If our frame of mind feeds only on the negative vibration, its own vibration will be gradually lowered. And when its vibration is lowered, it will create a much lowered vibration of the physical body. This lowered vibration of the physical body, will in turn be more prone to attracting the lower negative vibration of illness, and make the body more vulnerable to the sicknesses of the lower vibration bodies.

3. *Freedom from imbalance and death ideas*

Illness originates with the mind. It begins when one's mind convinces them that they are sick. When this happens there might not even be a doctor in the world to try and convince them otherwise. Only they can prove to themselves that they are actually totally fine and that there's absolutely nothing wrong with them whatsoever. In its most extreme cases a person, any person, is actually capable of literally depressing their body and mind from such thoughts or ideas to such an extent that they are actually known to be capable of quickly withering and dying.

One story I recall in particular years ago that seemed obvious at the time, but which I was later to confirm for myself, was not unique by any stretch of the imagination. It dealt with a patient in a hospital. After getting through the surgery, a patient accidentally overheard the surgeon discussing the results of the surgery as very depressing and hopeless. Things were so bad that the surgeon decided that it was better to hold off any treatment. Upon overhearing the news, a patient saw a complete reversal in their recovery. Their mood changed from that of hope to complete devastation. They had no appetite for anyone or anything, and could not stomach any further medication or prescribed treatments. What's the use? They felt it was pointless anyways. In response, the physicians couldn't understand how a routine surgery could cause these complications. A patient rapidly turned downhill and their symptoms worsened by the minute. The situation became all but completely hopeless, until it was found out that the surgeons in the hallway were discussing their pet dog. There's really no reason to recite any more of like and similar stories, because there's just so many of them. Like for example, when a student who died the next day after being told by all of her classmates that she looked terribly ill. As it turned out, they were only playing a prank to prove a mind over matter experiment.

The mind plays a leading role in an illness. Just think of how many times you were told some horrible news, did you have an excellent appetite for doing something exciting that day? Well, so much less are the people who experience pain and unpleasant symptoms at the onset of illness. And this is all at a times when they most need their energy for healing. They feel they haven't any strength left. And all they do is constantly repeat to themselves that their illness will end up confirming their doctor's worst predictions… Death.

For the average person the ideas of death and sickness are confirmed and reaffirmed on almost daily basis. When it comes to aging and death none of us are immune to the self-damage caused by these ideas. From the time the child is young enough to understand they are told that they are going to die. And they are coached to expect the inevitable symptoms as they age. Wrinkles, white hair, general weakening, they are told, are totally normal. And that they should just accept it as a part of the normal world. It's normal simply because they've accepted this as a fact.

4. *Letting go of fear*

Fear originates with a memory that isn't pleasant. At its strongest form it causes a panic attack and a physical shock. While at its milder form the fear turns into hatred, and milder still, into disgust.

Somewhere in the past the victim of fear had stored a memory in which they faced a situation they couldn't resolve. And because they couldn't or didn't have the preparation to understand what was going on to find ways to resolve it, it remained as a memory of an unresolved situation. Later, when they face a similar situation, the unresolved memory is reactivated. And transforms itself into what is known as the physical reaction (feeling) of fear. When the victim of fear experiences the physical reaction (emotion) of fear their focus and concentration is taken away from resolving the situation. And if they again do not resolve their unresolved memory, they will continue to experience the physical effects of fear.

Any thought form is a vibration that can be used by a person's frame of mind in order to set the operational vibration for the rest of the physical body. This process goes like this, a person's frame of mind is set up by the thought forms which it accepts or repels. The kind of thought forms which a frame of mind accepts or repels is determined by how closely its vibration matches with the overall vibration of their frame of mind. If a thought form has a matching vibration to the frame of mind, it is accepted. And if not, it is repelled. Likewise, the overall vibration of a person's frame of mind is also determined by the vibration of the kind of thought forms which happen to dominate their frame of mind. If the frame of mind is nourished by lower (heavy) vibration thought forms, its overall vibration is likewise lowered. If, on the other hand, it's nourished by positive (higher) vibration thoughts, then the overall vibration of the frame of mind is also increased and the positive (light) physical effects on the body are created.

This whole thought cycle begins to conclude when the overall vibration of the thoughts and the frame of mind reach the same level. When this happens the frame of mind is then ready to set the operational vibration rate for the rest of the physical body. So that the thoughts, the frame of mind and the physical body all operate at the same vibration. In the thought cycle of an unresolved memory a person has a thought of an unresolved memory. This can also be called the 'worse fears are realized' thought vibration. In this process the thought form of an unresolved memory has a vibration of an unresolved situation thought form. When this thought form of an unresolved situation enters the frame of mind, its vibration sets the overall vibration of the frame of mind. Then, once the overall vibration of their frame of mind is set at that level, it then sets a lower operational vibration for the physical body. Because like attracts like, the vibration of their physical body reaches the same lower level as their thoughts. The vibration of an unresolved memory is turned into the physical reaction of fear. And they physically feel the vibrations of their heavy thoughts.

This is because when the memory of an unpleasant situation from the past is accepted by the frame of mind, it doesn't have the memory of solution. That unresolved situation had never been resolved and a person encountering it again has no set of solutions to work with. They again encounter the same unpleasant situation from the past, and again feel powerless to do anything to resolve it. The physical effect of this unresolved memory is compounded by the lowered physical vibration which matches the overall vibration of the unresolved memory thought form. Like attracts like, which means the thoughts, the frame of mind and the physical body all reach the same vibration. When the body operates at the vibration of the unresolved memory thought form the physical body experiences a physical paralysis. And in an extreme case cause them to feel a panic attack. A memory with a clear resolution, however, has a different thought vibration and therefore causes the physical body to experience a different physical vibration.

For the thought cycle of fear to be broken, one must reconstruct their unresolved memory. The unresolved memory has to become a resolved memory. When they find the solution the vibration of the unresolved memory thought form will be raised to the vibration of the resolved memory thought form. This will also cause the overall vibration of the physical response to be raised to another level. When the thought of a same situation is restored in their memory as being resolved, its vibration will no longer trigger the physical reaction of fear. A person will be familiar with a solution of how to resolve a similar situation should it arise again, and won't feel frightened by it again.

5. Resolving pain and
Resolving the kind of pain that's a manageable annoyance

Pain is a thought. And like every thought that enters a person's frame of mind, it's ultimately there by choice. This means that a person ultimately has control over it and can ultimately choose whether or not to accept it or repel it from their frame of mind.

Basically, the pain is a thought (thought form) that enters a person's frame of mind. Once there, the pain thought form can be triggered over and over again. When this thought is triggered, it becomes activated and a person experiences the physical reaction of pain, which can range the scale from minor annoyance to something dramatic. This process basically starts with the trigger. This trigger reactivates the thought of pain in a person's frame of mind. Sometimes, the trigger just allows the thought of pain to enter their frame of mind and stay there. Once, the thought of pain becomes active it can then begin to dominate a person's frame of mind. Then, when the thought of pain dominates a person's frame of mind, a person's frame of mind then takes on the overall vibration of those thoughts. As like attracts like, the lowered vibration of their frame of mind will cause it to accept the thought forms of similar vibration. In the case of the thought of pain, this will cause a person to accept other thoughts of pain.

This process of thought manifestation continues after the

overall vibration of a person's thought forms sets the overall operational vibration for their frame of mind, and they reach an identical level. When this happens, then the overall vibration of the frame of mind can set up the overall operational vibration for the rest of the physical body. So that when the overall vibration of their thought forms, their frame of mind and their physical vibration reach the same lower level, then the vibration of the thought form of pain will become manifested in the vibration of the physical body. Their physical body will then operate at the vibrational level of the thought form of pain, and a person will experience this lowered vibration on their physical body as the physical reaction (pain).

To stop the physical reaction of pain from becoming manifested, a person must repel the thought form of pain that causes that physical reaction. They have to interrupt the pain thought cycle from becoming manifested in their physical vibration. If the degree of physical pain is very severe, this will not be a quick fix. This is because, the severity of the physical reaction of pain indicates the level at which this thought has come to dominate their frame of mind.

If a person can recognize that their frame of mind is dominated by the thoughts of pain, then they have their work cut out for them. At first they can begin to gradually introduce the thought forms of higher (positive) vibration. When more of the lighter thoughts are accepted by their frame of mind, this will reduce the amount of thoughts of pain in their frame of mind. Then, when more of the positive thought forms are accepted by a person's frame of mind, its overall vibration will begin to increase. The increased vibration of their thought forms will cause the overall vibration of their frame of mind to lighten up, and accept the thoughts of higher vibration. The lighter vibration of their frame of mind will also determine what kind of thought forms it will accept and which ones it will repel. So, with the increased vibration, their frame of mind will accept the thought forms of matching vibration, and repel the thought forms which do not match the overall vibration of their frame of mind. This means that the lower (heavier) thoughts of the pain will not be accepted. And their dominance in a person's frame of mind will be reduced.

This thought cycle manifestation of lighter thoughts will be completed when the overall operational vibration of their physical body will match the overall operational vibration of their frame of mind. This will happen because when the overall vibration of their thought forms and their frame of mind reach the same lighter level of vibration, then their frame of mind will then be able to set the overall operational vibration of the rest of the physical body to the same higher level. As this happens, the thought cycle manifestation process will be completed. Their overall thought forms, their overall frame of mind, and the physical body will operate at the same higher vibration. And when their physical body will operate at a lighter vibration, a person's physical reaction to their thoughts will likewise be changed, and their former irritation will be gone.

6. *Becoming a little child*

If adulthood is your fantasy when you are a child, then childhood is really an ideal of most people's lives. It's usually marked by the best health they'll ever have and the remarkable demonstrations of healing. This is an ideal and there's no reason why it shouldn't be this way for everyone.

It's fair to say that for most people childhood is looked on as the once carefree time in which they ran around, played games and didn't suffer their life's biggest imbalances that are to come much, much later. At this wonderful time, health-wise speaking, their entire life energy is dedicated to the growth of their body, to absorbing all of the newness of life and looking for new and exciting games to play. Because of this, and how extremely busy they are, most children really haven't much time or energy left to spend on destabilizing their body and mind. Just when it appears the new or exotic illness is about to set in, by and large, they are somehow able to spurt out of it. They really waste no time on not being able to pursue what they really love, and only what they love. The miracle of childhood is in the miraculous ability to heal. This remarkable ability to heal at a moment's notice is what has endeared all children to their older counterparts, who seem to have all those things in reverse.

What does it mean to be healed? It means the old cells are replaced, or recycled in order to give way to, you guessed it, the cells of a child, or one's younger cells. When you get a scrape on your knee, what happens? The 'older' layer of skin is scraped off and the brand new, young, rejuvenated cells take their place, until they become completely healed and restored. Well, this same process continues naturally and always with the rest of the body just as surely as it does with a small scrape or a scab. If it didn't happen the cells wouldn't regenerate in time and the physical healing would be impossible.

Everything in the body, or at least most of it, gets replaced with newer and younger cells all the time. This is a natural function of the body that has been long publicized by many researchers in the area of rejuvenation. Without this natural rejuvenation of the body and mind no life would be possible. The physical body needs rejuvenation and is in a constant state of replacing the older with the younger cells. If the skin, hair, or muscles cells weren't regularly replaced with younger cells, the physical body would be riddled with holes and be completely unable to heal. This goes for everyone, including the people who look 'older'.

In actual fact, a vast majority of human cells are nowhere as old as could be suggested. And have plenty of young cells to speak of. The human body goes through cycles of regeneration on average about every several years in which it gets completely replaced. This process happens at a miniscule level, cell by cell, hair by hair, fiber by fiber, nerve ending by nerve ending. All this means is that at any given moment in time there may not even be a person older than about ten years old. Some people look older because the younger cells fill the already assigned spaces. So, if there was a scar, a wrinkle or a stretch mark, it will remain a scar, a wrinkle or stretch mark even though the skin cells that make it still happen to be very young. This happens even in very young children. But to a degree even the reality of old wounds had been demonstrated to be transcended.

7. *Prayer*

To be effective, the healing prayer needs to offer at least these things.

1. The prayer must relax the body to open the flow for healing.

2. It must retain these exact same or better results each and every time it's called upon by its practitioner.

3. It must be sufficient enough to divert its practitioner's attention and energy away from their illness and onto healing. While also excluding anything and everything that doesn't happen to match the healing objective.

4. It must enable its practitioner to see, feel, and sense in every way possible that they are fully capable of healing and are healing. Their prayer must convince them beyond the least shadow of a doubt that their desired healing is as good as, or is in fact completely achieved.

If these basic and fundamental parameters are met or exceeded, the prayer will heal.

1. When one's body and mind are sufficiently relaxed and rested, the internal flow, so vital to the supply of energy and nutrients to the areas especially affected by an illness, is normalized. This happens naturally when the body is left enough alone to do so. But any stress and tension during an illness puts additional demand on the body's depleted energy

reserves. This interference with the body's normal flow functions diverts its much needed attention and energy, away from only being used to heal.

For the healing to take place the physical attention and energy must not be spent on maintaining the same stress and tension. So, if the prayer is going to do anything fast, it must relax a person enough to open their body to receive healing. When they become unshackled their attention and energy is freed to restore nutrients to the affected area.

2. It's simply not enough for a prayer to convince someone that they are healing only once. A prayer should not leave them stranded with negative thoughts such as anger, hatred, worry, anxiety, fear, misery, as well as hopelessness of being able to achieve their desired level of health. Such thoughts would again tense and close up the body. If the prayer lets a person down like this, it may be harder for a person to make another effort at healing.

3. At the sign of any healing one begins to spend less of their energy on their illness and more on what they actually enjoy doing. This is because when one is able to place all of their attention and energy on only their healing, they inevitably bring themselves closer toward their achievement of their desired level of health. The easiest way to understand this is that when one is able to put all their attention and energy on achieving their healing, they are that much more likely to achieve it. And a prayer should do this too.

4. When the prayer allows its practitioner to place their

attention and energy on only their desired healing, that healing will become more real. And when this healing is sensed in every way possible it will become real. And when it becomes real the practitioner will see, feel and sense in every way possible that they are indeed healing.

Another way to understand this is that a prayer is ultimately just a thought that has its own vibration. And the healing, likewise, is also a thought that has its vibration. This means that when we pray, we place the vibration of that prayer thought into our frame of mind. If our prayer is healing, it has a higher vibration and therefore results in the raising of the overall vibration of the frame of mind. Then, once the overall vibration of the frame of mind is raised, it then sets the operational vibration for the rest of the body. Then, when the overall physical vibration matches the overall vibration of healing, it causes the physical body to experience the reality of that higher vibration. This is why how we think (pray) is important for the overall operation of the physical body.

8. Prayers collection/Prayers reception

This world of ours is so full of wonderful prayers of people for not just their family and friends, but for all people all over the world and their health and optimal healing. These prayers speak to the universal communities of the undeniable kindness of the members of the human race toward one another. Prayers for the strangers they've never met, but with whom they believe, no matter the distance, they share an undeniable bond of their extended human family.

I've seen and heard, and personally participated on many prayer occasions, and I'm sure you did too. They are made up of people from all walks of life, beliefs and religions. Whether these prayers are spoken by Buddhists, Hindus, Christians, Muslims, Spiritualists, Non-religious, or whatever else, their prayers are all dedicated, among other things, to the optimal healing of all those who are in need of healing.

I was privileged to watch these mass prayers broadcast on television. I have also read and heard about specific groups in many cities around the world who meet under various flags every day, or on specific days of the week with a sole purpose of sending out those prayers of healing to those who need healing. These collective prayers are specifically included in the regular services of various congregations and are prayed with the intent of reaching those who need them. Sometimes they are intended for specific types of illnesses, but more often than not, the prayers are sent out just for the sake of whatever illness one desires to heal, to persons unknown.

These prayers are important to help people recover because they provide the vital energy that can then be consciously tapped into to achieve healing. The energy from these prayers, just like any other energy, has a tremendous ability to enable its recipient to heal.

Despite this, many people still feel that there isn't anyone in the whole wide world who even cares enough about them to pray. In their feeling of isolation they have less reason to be motivated and inspired to heal. Instead of feeling comforted in the darkest hour by the idea that someone cares, they feel the exact opposite. They feel panic, anger, fear, resentment, hatred, anxiety, worry, misery or a sense of complete hopelessness that they will ever be able to heal. And, so, while on its end the healing energy may still be enough to help that person eventually heal, its powerful influence remains greatly curtailed due to their noncooperation.

Without the free will it will make it that much harder for the healing energy to smash its way through the personal defenses of negativity. These heavy thoughts will actually block that energy from being able to break through to their illness.

9. Communication/Conversation with affected area

If it's indeed true that there's a purpose to everything in the universe and that everything is there for a reason. Then it's certainly not a stretch to suppose that an illness also has a purpose. This reason goes far beyond some elaborate scheme to somehow punish a person for their prior misdeeds. Its purpose for being there is to impart an important lesson, or message, to be learned by that individual. The healing, therefore, rests in figuring out the message behind the existence of an illness.

Ultimately, it isn't at all true that the only purpose for the presence of these illnesses is to cause an illness. They are there to fulfill a far more elaborate role than we might imagine: their own all important mission in life. And it doesn't include causing an illness anymore than the purpose of a human life is to simply rob, murder, exploit or enslave. A human fulfills their own purpose to exist, just as well as an illness, while committing their negative things.

Every cell that is alive represents a sentient being and is therefore full of consciousness. And while it may not be the kind of consciousness an average person would be able to recognize right away, each living cell of the body and mind possesses intelligence and consciousness. The consciousness of each and every cell, virus, bacteria or a deformed cell, isn't exactly the same as that of animals and people. Their consciousness is different and uses different modes of communication. The virus, bacteria, or a deformed cell, does not, per say, wants to get a job in order to get cash in order to go to the store in order to buy food in order to make friends. But, then, those viruses, bacteria, and deformed cells really don't have to have the exact same consciousness as a human in order to be valid. Their consciousness is different because their purposes for being alive are also different.

Just because some creature is disagreeable to somebody based on its appearance or little understood function doesn't mean that that creature doesn't have a life and has its own important purpose to fulfill. This purpose can sometimes be as simple as passing on a lesson or a message to their more evolved cousin. The viruses, bacteria and deformed cells are not ill in themselves per say simply because their presence appears to cause the imbalance. They are ultimately spiritual (soul endowed) creatures, who learn to react or adapt accordingly to their environment. And their purpose for being in the physical body will be fulfilled at any time their message is figured out by the recipient (aka the sick person). When it happens, an illness has no further reason to remain, and can then move on with the greater evolutionary plan for their spirit.

Everything needs a purpose to exist. And without some purpose for existing nothing can exist any further. Illnesses are there to fulfill their important life's role and to move on. As spiritual beings they don't always want to be a virus, bacteria, or a deformed cell. They want to have a chance to develop and mature spiritually in their own way. They don't want to have to come back over and over again to bring more misery or be fought with at every chance. Once their desperate lesson is properly communicated they can then be free to move on. And sometimes their message deserves to be heard.

10. *Loving kindness to the affected part of the body*

Without a doubt, loving kindness is the most creative and potent force in the universe that there is. Those who know of its tremendous capacity believe that it is a force behind every achievement of the human race, including, undoubtedly, the physical healing. No matter how unbelievable or impossible something sounds at first, anything's possible if the force and power of loving kindness are behind it. This force is evident in every achievement, every building, every accumulation of anything, and every relationship and indeed the very procreation of the human race undoubtedly depends on it.

When someone feels loving kindness toward something, that something always becomes that much easier to achieve. If one loves ice cream there is more of a chance one will eat it; if one loves money, there is more of a chance one will seek to possess it, etc. When someone has a lover, a friend, a family, or someone they adore, then it really won't matter what anybody has to say to have them feel otherwise. So, no matter what is said about them in order to reverse their feelings toward them, they will still feel love and kindness toward them. Or, what if that something happens to be their possession, job, a pet, a personal item, or a wish, would those be treated any differently. Here again, no matter what, they will still continue to feel loving kindness toward those things simply because those things cause them to experience a whole array of wonderful and pleasant emotions which make them feel good. And when one hates and feels angry at something, they are that much less likely to achieve it.

Have you ever met a person whose only purpose to heal is to become more hateful, angrier, bitter, anxious, frustrated, miserable, desperate or utterly hopeless of ever being able to achieve their desired level of health? Isn't it actually very often the exact reverse? When people feel negative probably the last thing on their mind is healing. When they feel negative they fall ill. Then, when they fall ill, the average person feels they have more reasons to feel negative. But getting rid of negative emotions always results in healing. And one of the first signs of healing is the replacement of the negative emotions for the positive.

11. Crystal ball

In order to stay healthy a person has to be able to protect themselves from anything that can cause illness. And in order to heal a person has to be able to keep an illness from reentering their body. This means that their physical body must be quarantined from any cause of illness long enough to allow it to heal itself. All this sounds really simple. But in the real world things never turn out quite as simple as one hoped.

Despite one's best efforts at trying to stay healthy by doing what one possibly can in order to protect themselves from the causes of illness, there can still be some accidental situations when one can still get exposed. Perhaps it might be something they ate at a restaurant, or it may come through a negative person. Whatever the causes, it's clear that in this world there's no surest way to ensure that anyone won't ever get sick. There are also no surest ways to always keep one's causes of their illness at bay. A sick person can still do what they possibly can to protect themselves from illness triggers and still have accidental exposures to illness triggers.

If the human body is so vulnerable to the causes of illness, then what can be done to stay healthy? The seemingly simple solution to this quarantine is in the power of the human mind. The same mind that has both the ability to sicken and to heal.

This power of the mind is enhanced when it has a clear idea of what it intends to do in order to focus its attention and energy. The reason for this ability of the human mind to crystallize and focus its ideas is biological. Our bodies have the properties of a crystal. The human DNA, and therefore every cell of the human body, is crystalline in nature. Of course, let's note that its consistency isn't the same as the stone crystals. But, the crystalline structure of the entire human body is, albeit, in its softer, less denser form, nevertheless just as naturally occurring as any crystal. Without dwelling on the modern science that proves it to be definitively so, the easiest thing anyone can do is to pick a strand of human hair and compare its structure to that of a naturally occurring rock crystals, or soft fiber optics, which are also designed to take advantage of the crystalline structure. Looking at the long shaft of hair you will see how it glows, how pliable it is, and how translucent it is. This endless variety of the human crystal is also found in the structures of bones, eye lenses, and nails.

The biological properties of a human body lend themselves naturally to being able to heal when one has a crystal clear idea to do so. This happens when one's mind is able to use its natural human crystal structure to focus its attention and energy on their desired healing. Once the intent of a human mind becomes undisputedly crystal clear then a person can strategically place their attention and energy on what it is they want. For example, if one's mental intent is to surround themselves with a layer of protection in order to heal, then their human crystal structure can further magnify their clear intent.

This is where the visualization of a crystal ball lends itself naturally when it comes to the achievement of the protection that the body needs to get healthy. It's easy to visualize and at the same time is simple enough to allow the mind to have a framework in which it can place its healing intent. For some it may be a pyramid, for some an octahedron, a dipyramid, a bicone or any other polyhedra they are comfortable with. For some that polyhedron may be revolving at a particular speed and direction. Or, even have a particular tinge, or an inner or outer glow, if they so prefer. Whatever it is, one must keep in mind that a crystal clear shape is possible as a result of their crystal clear intent of protecting their body and mind from illness. That crystal clear intention has to come first.

12. Conversation with the Higher self/
Higher consciousness on perceived lessons

The human body and mind are governed and managed from 'above' by one's spirit, or higher consciousness. This higher-self uses the human body and mind so long as it can enable it to go about achieving its desired life goals. All it means is that healing is impossible without the prior approval, or a go ahead from one's higher mind.

It would behoove anyone to communicate with their higher consciousness (soul) for the healing advice. The opposite is often the case with the average person. Usually, when they want to heal the first thing they do is go and talk it over with their friend, their family, or a professional. So long as that somebody isn't them it's pretty much okay to be advised. Sometimes a person goes and searches a world over in order to find a way to get healthy, while never giving themselves the meaningful opportunity to talk to 'themselves'. They leave 'themselves' out of their own health decisions. To go on like this is to ignore the inherent power and ability to achieve anything within. Their spirit possesses tremendous power, knowledge and resourcefulness.

Experiments with subjects under hypnosis (a type of trance) have sufficiently demonstrated that the human being ultimately has an access to unlimited supply of knowledge. Many subjects have been asked under hypnosis to find the solution to the most impossible type of information and retrieved it with ease. Miraculous people like Edgar Cayce, Wolf Messing, and others, have amazed doctors with their uncanny ability to access the spiritual, or Akashik, records. They not only precisely located the area of illness and its source, but also the simple way to cure it. Other pioneering authors have done their search for the truth with hypnosis. Among them are Michael Newton, Brian Weiss and Dolores Cannon. She had spent decades proving to people that the source of an illness is often found in one's past life. And she used hypnosis to search out the past lives in order to find the origin of the illness. And when that answer wasn't shown there, she went directly to the 'SC', or a person's 'subconscious'. Once the purpose for an illness is understood and addressed, then a person finds healing.

Each person also has a personal access to their higher self by many means other than a psychic or a hypnotist. Everyone can find healing by reaching their higher self for the healing advice. The access to their own healing records, according to Edgar Cayce or Dolores Cannon, is always available to every single person alive. And as it so happens, each person always taps into that knowledge (their spirit knowledge) without the awareness of having done so. Some of the common ways in which the communication comes is through premonition, a gut feeling, a dream or an intuition. Every time someone takes the right turn in the road or heeds some warning deep within, they communicate with their higher self.

In the same way that the architect communicates with the building, so likewise one's spirit uses its human body to communicate its message to its recipient. These intended messages can and often do come through an illness. An illness is used by one's spirit to communicate a particular message. And this message often comes in the symbolic form of an illness. In her groundbreaking book, *The Soul Speak*, Julia Cannon tells that once the message behind an illness is understood and fully addressed, then a person will find healing. When their intended message is learned a person can move to other things.

Ultimately, one's higher self always knows best when it comes to healing an illness. Behind each of our bodies is a spiritual being, who uses the body and mind in order to make our spiritual, and or inter-dimensional experience that much more enriching. We have those truly boundless spirits to guide us to healing. We just have to communicate with them.

13. Identifying with self in the future tense/
Imbalance is temporary

No matter how difficult it is to be ill it will never always be that way. Eventually, and inevitably everyone will feel balanced and well again. One will always be young and healthy again, and will always have a chance, if they so choose, to pick up again right where they've left off. To begin to understand how that's possible we must depart from the narrow interpretation of time that it is only a chronological sequence of events. It is an interconnected whole. This interconnected substance of time can also be likened to the 'string of time'.

Time isn't some broken up string that marks the separation of distant events. Time binds these events together. And because each of the events is a part of the whole, they are said to be happening simultaneously and at the same time. This broader understanding of time means that we are actually both in the future, the present and the past all at the same time. So, unlike the narrower interpretation of time, the broader interpretation suggests that the events such as health and illness aren't islands separated by vast ocean miles. They are interconnected parts of the whole.

All of the events on the necklace of time are interconnected, and every event in time is a part of the whole. This means that wherever you might be on your string of time, whatever event you might be experiencing, you're likewise simultaneously experiencing all of the other events. This means that if someone is experiencing an illness, then they likewise have the ability to experience healing. Their healing is already a part of the whole timeline. And since they are already experiencing all of their events simultaneously (or now), then they can also choose which event in time they would rather focus on and then go for it. Would they rather experience their healing now, or wait for later. Whatever decision they will have made, it is already a part of the necklace of time and can be experienced as much as they want to.

The interconnectedness of time (the string of time) means that the 'time' that separates the past and the future is so imperceptible that it almost doesn't exist. One split second you're in the past, the next you're in the future, and so on. But how exactly can you use the interconnectedness of time to get from experiencing (focusing on) illness to experiencing healing? This is brought about by the degree in which you place yourself in the healing future.

How well you can experience that future with your senses as that 'future' (healing) is happening determines how quickly you can transition on the string of time from the event of illness to the event of healing. For example, suppose you're about to go and shake your friend's hand. As you rapidly walk toward them, it gets to the point that both of your hands are extended to one another until the future of shaking each other's hands becomes a reality. When this happens, you will have effectively, and for a brief moment, entered the future. The moment right before you're both about to shake hands would represent the relative clarity with which you observe that future. Then, at the moment that the future of shaking hands happens, you will see, feel and sense it in every way possible in such a way that you would be literally touching that 'future' into existence.

What is important to take away from this is that the relative certainty of one's future of ultimate healing is determined by the clarity with which one sees their healing. And just like with the handshake example, one's relative view of their future of healing is what literally defines and determines what they see, feel and sense in their present. Right before their healing future happens the clarity with which that person sees it, feels it, and senses it in every way possible is dramatically increased. And what might have only a moment ago been seen as just a 'hazy' vision of the future, now becomes a crystal clear reality.

14. Healing visualization

We see (visualize) things all the time. The downside of it is that usually our vision becomes very biased and we see what we want to see, and often neglect to see what we don't want to see. We see what we expect to see and don't see what we don't know exists.

We use the visualization skills all the time in our mind whether we know it or not. And the mind of the average person is constantly busy with visualizing things all the time. Even when we sleep we also see different visions in our mind in the form of dreams.

We are very visual creatures and this ability helps us to get what we want. We window-shop and we watch television and read. When we can see something we get a better idea of what it is we want and find better ways to change things. We use this skill to study and to create things. And we apply our visualization skill set to get what we want and to move away from what we don't want.

When we want something we are more likely to get attracted to it, or attract it to ourselves. And when we don't want something we are more likely to be repelled from it, or repel it from ourselves. So that when we want something, and have a clear idea of what it is we are aiming for, we are then able to focus and concentrate our energy on obtaining it. Conversely, when we don't want something, and have a clear idea of what it is we are trying to avoid, we are then able to focus and concentrate our energy away from it.

In basic sense, the reason visualization works so well for us is because it enables us to focus and concentrate our thinking on something. And when our thinking is focused and concentrated on something it sets the overall vibration for the kinds of thoughts we are likely to receive. Like attracts like. Like energy attracts like energy. Like thoughts attract like thoughts. And like vibration attracts like vibrations.

When the thoughts that come into our mind are of a similar vibration, they then set the overall vibration for our frame of mind. This is because the thoughts in our mind are like nourishment for our frame of mind. When our frame of mind is composed of matching thought vibrations, these then instruct the rest of the frame of mind how to operate. And as like attracts like, the prevalence of these thought vibrations will then set the overall vibration of our entire frame of mind. Then, once the vibration of our frame of mind is set up, our frame of mind then tunes the rest of the body to operate (vibrate) at our chosen vibration. So, that when our thoughts, our frame of mind, and our body reach the same vibration, they are said to be operating at the matching vibration and this exchange cycle is complete. This type of process happens all the time, and it determines at what vibration our physical body will operate.

For example, if our thoughts focus on illness, they are said to be of negative (lower) vibration. When we have enough of these lower thought vibrations, they then determine the overall vibration of our frame of mind. So that, when our thinking is predominated with lower (heavy) thought vibrations, then the overall vibration of our frame of mind will also be lowered. Then, when our frame of mind operates at a lower vibration, it then instructs the body to likewise begin to operate at a lower (heavier) vibration. And when our thoughts, our frame of mind and our physical body operate at a lower vibration, our physical body will attract illness, because it matches that heavy vibration. It will mean that it will be harder for us to attract the healing (or the higher positive vibration).

If you understand all this then you can see the potential impact our visualization can have on our physical bodies. If you want health (or higher positive vibrations), then you must be more responsible about how you use your visualization skills. But if all you see in your mind is illness, then you shouldn't be surprised that it will be harder for your physical body to heal. You have to adjust your thinking and make sure you visualize the thoughts with the vibration you want. If you visualize (or focus and concentrate) on the thoughts of healing, then the vibration of your thoughts and your frame of mind will be raised. And when the vibration of your frame of mind becomes positive, your physical body will raise its vibration in order to operate in sync with your frame of mind. Then, when the vibration of your thoughts, your mind and your body matches, then your body will attracts the similar lighter and positive vibrations of healing.

15. Cosmic rain shower of light visualization

Our entire world is imbued with energy that goes largely unnoticed to the average people. This energy is responsible for everything that goes on in the entire universe, from the smallest atom to the largest super galaxies and beyond. This energy of light rains down on earth always and forever. It is what is responsible for the creation of life on this planet, everything that's on it, in it and of it as dealing with the material (physical) matter of existence. Like any conscious intelligence in the universe it's eager to tune in and give extra help where it can.

This energy is different however from the solar light, solar radiation, or any kind of radiation, period. It is beyond our sun, our view of the solar radiation and other radiation. Any radiation is a natural byproduct of the functioning of every matter. Superseding this, and imbuing all, is the cosmic rain shower of this energy. It is responsible for the life and health of every creature. Without the generous and continuous presence of this cosmic energy the healing of our physical bodies would be without fuel. It's true to say that at this moment in our human history this energy is beyond the comprehension of mere mortals and the most advanced scientist alike. And this might probably remain so for now.

And yet, we know enough to be certain that this cosmic energy rains down on each and every one of us in copious amounts, and uninterrupted torrents each and every single moment of our existence. It literally permeates every single matter known to exist. It doesn't matter if one is buried alive under miles of rock, or is a prisoner in the mechanized environment. What matters is that as long as we are alive we most necessarily tap into that energy to survive. From the smallest mite, to the largest specie alive, their current state of health and wellbeing wouldn't be possible without this energy. And to most people this energy is totally invisible.

The cosmic energy is conscious and intelligent. And has the wherewithal to resonate more strongly with those people who are aware enough to recognize its existence. It isn't to say that somehow this energy is transformed and becomes something other than itself when one consciously communicates with it. No, it remains unchanged. The only difference is that when it's reached out to on a conscious level it has the built-in ability to consciously respond back. It's like it's given a greater permission to more actively participate and interact with the human body. When the permission is granted then the human consciousness and the higher consciousness can connect to cooperate to achieve healing.

The conscious cooperation with this energy is especially enhanced through the visual images. To understand this it helps to realize that not everything can communicate with words or writing like humans. This is why any visualization becomes a great tool to bridge the communication gap with other intelligences. An example of this would be when one is able to visualize how this cosmic energy continuously washes over their physical body. This visualization is simple enough to activate the conscious commutation with that energy. When one establishes this communication then the intelligence of the cosmic rain shower of light has the permission to better tune to the individual's physical needs. Conversely, if one is unwilling to communicate with that energy, the higher consciousness will respond in kind and will not violate the sanctity of one's free will to choose what they want. It'll just go about its business and not bother that person more than is necessary to nourish them.

16. White light of protection and cleansing

Physical protection form illness and cleansing are very important to the overall healing process. And the healing depends on how well the body is able to protect and cleanse itself from the causes of illness. How this process actually takes place is important.

To the surprise of the average person, the healing actually never begins with the physical body, but is often the consequence of whether or not a person is able to protect and cleanse themselves from the source of illness. This means that in order to truly protect and to cleanse the body from an illness it makes no sense to try and address the bare surface of what's actually going on. Instead it makes better sense to understand the source of both the healing and the illness itself. Once the deeper processes are understood they can then be applied for more permanent healing results.

To begin to understand how the physical protection and cleansing from an illness actually works, is to understand a fundamental reality of nature. This reality points to the fact that both an illness and the physical body have a particular wavelength (a vibration) at which they both resonate. We call this vibration a thought form. A thought form can have either a lower or a higher vibration. Sometimes we refer to the lower vibration as a heavy (negative) vibration, and the higher vibration as a light (positive) vibration.

When we look at the physical illness, it's usually known as the lower (negative) vibration. This means that an illness is considered a lower (negative) thought form. So, for example if the body is prone to illness or has an illness, that body is considered to be operating at a lower (negative) vibration. Like attracts like. This means that if a person thinks that they are ill or has thoughts that are negative (heavy) in nature they will be more likely to attract illness, and less likely to heal. Again, everything attracts like vibrations. Negative thoughts attract negative thoughts. And lower vibrations resonate with the lower vibrations.

Now that we understand how negativity attracts illness we can briefly look at the process of how someone becomes ill based on these observations. An illness begins not on the physical level, but on a thought level. An illness itself, just like anything else, is just a vibration (a thought form). Basically, that's really all it is. If a person's mind predominates with negative thoughts and they are not accepting positive thoughts, the overall vibration of their frame of mind will be lowered. Then, when the vibration of their frame of mind is lowered, they will be more likely to accept the negative thoughts and repel the positive thoughts. Like attracts like, and so after a while the lowered vibration of their frame of mind will result in the lowered vibration of the physical body. So that eventually, their thoughts, their frame of mind and their physical body will operate at the same vibration. And, so, since an illness is represented by a lower vibration it will be more attracted to the physical body that operates at a similar resonance.

The white light on the other hand, is a very positive (light) thought form, and operates at a higher vibration. And this makes it unique when it comes to increasing the vibration of the physical body. It's very straight forward and can be easily pictured.

You see, every thought form in the universe has a purpose and each though form operates at its own distinct and subtle vibration. Every thought form is like that, and that's why every material (physical) item has its purpose and is uniquely suited to the task it's assigned to for. Nothing is wasted in the universe, not even a thought, and everything has a purpose. If we can understand this we can find a good illustration of this concept in the physical world in the seven colors of the rainbow: Red, Orange, Yellow, Green, Blue, Indigo, Violet. As you look at each color, you can clearly see that each is very unique and is really unlike the others. Further still, each color operates at its own unique vibration for which it is best suited.

The color white is unique in that it's not found in the rainbow of the seven colors. The reason for that is because it's considered a higher vibration color. Its properties are those of protection and cleansing. And the physical properties of the color white background show any blemishes or discoloration.

Another property of the color white is that it's very easy to picture and recognize. This makes it a very easy target vibration thought form. Visualizing it (thinking it) doesn't really require much and can be easily done. This means that one can quickly raise the overall vibration of their frame of mind to that resonance. Just by visualizing the color white, one's thoughts are instantly raised to that vibration level. Then, when the thoughts are raised to a particular vibration level, they in turn raise the overall vibration of the frame of mind. And, then, when the overall vibration of the frame of mind is raised, it then sets the vibration level for the rest of the physical body.

If, for example, the physical illness is represented by the thoughts of lower vibration, then this means that when a person's thoughts, their frame of mind and their physical body all operate at a higher vibration, their physical body will be less likely to attract the thought forms of the lower vibration. And will be more likely to attract the higher positive vibration. Like attracts like, and so the physical body will attract healing if its overall vibration is positive. And likewise, if its overall vibration is negative it will be less likely to attract healing. If this happens, the white light of protection and cleansing becomes very handy to quickly realign the vibration of one's physical body with the positive vibration of healing.

17. Rainbow light of cleansing and complete healing

Different parts of the human body are healed by different methods. The different methods have to be used because each part of the body is unique and has its own unique way of healing and functioning. And even though they are all parts of the same physical body as a whole, each organ and part of the body is still different. This means that in order to use healing properly the one doing the healing has to have a pretty good idea at how each part of the body functions and how it's healed.

One of the first things one can understand about the physical parts of the body is that they are all color-coded. Their color is important because it tells us the unique vibration at which each part of the body operates. When we know at what energetic vibration each part of the body operates, we can then use the known tools to help us reach that vibration, and restore health.

As it so happens, the colors of the rainbow and the parts of the body are closely similar. This is because the like colors have a similar energetic vibration. And each color of the rainbow has its own particular vibration (frequency) that corresponds to each part of the body. When the physical body is healthy, each part of the body has a good bright color. This indicates that everything's well and there is a 'chromatic' (energetic) balance in the physical body. Conversely, if the physical body is ill this would also show in the discoloration of the affected parts of the body. For example, the arm that turns purple from a particularly nasty bruise informs us that there is an excess of purple in that area. It then reminds us to 'mind' (color purple) what we are doing, or at least contemplate as to the reasons behind the possible causes.

Ultimately, whatever the overall natural complexion each person has, it must have an overall 'chromatic balance' in order to stay healthy. Likewise, each part of the body also has its own 'chromatic' (energetic) balance that must also be maintained if those parts are to remain healthy. Their unique blend of colors must be balanced and remain energetically vibrant.

Here are some of the basic color characteristics as they relate to the different body parts:

1. The Purple, or very rich dark blue, communicates the energy related to the brain matter and healthy mental functions.

2. The sky blue alludes to the air. It is important to the throat and lung area, and its vibration is important for breathing clearly.

3. The green is particularly effective in healing the heart, and is known for its calming effect.

4. Yellow is of the solar plexus area and resembles sunshine. It is greatly restoring of the nerves and the communication between them in the body.

5. Dark orange seems to associate with the gut. When the gut is imbalanced it will bring attention to itself with vibrant orange.

6. Very rich red, or scarlet color, is more suited to the conditions invigorating the blood flow and the vitality of libido.

7. The white insures that each part of the body is connected with one another and that they smoothly communicate with each other. The clarity of this color is signified by the eyes or the overall clear complexion of one's body and mind when all is balanced and healthy.

The physical body is chromatic. And each bodily part necessitates its own particular gamut (combination) of colors. The easiest way to understand this is to see that each color of the rainbow would be impossible without the other colors which help make each one of them up. So, blue and yellow make green, orange and green make yellow, and so on and so forth. Likewise, even though each area of the body and mind is dominated by its own particular hormone, or admixture, which give it its chromatic (colorful) expression. Each part of the body still meets its own unique needs by relying on the rest of the body. This process is properly described as a biological and bodily network which has its own proper supply and communication channels with one another. The heart, for example, pumps blood to every area of the body, while the lungs supply the oxygen to each and every cell. The brain sends the signals they can all use, while the sex organs pump the entire body and mind for action. So on and so forth.

In their balanced state these colors completely immerse each and every part of the physical body. And in turn, the body parts readily accept and absorb their particular combination of divine colors which best fit with their optimal health. So, for example, one's head might have too much coolness of the dark blue, but not the sufficient amount of green in order to sufficiently relax and not overdo. By contrast, the veins show up as blue, because the blood within them has been cut off from the oxygen and so travels back to the lungs in order to re-oxygenate with a fresh supply of oxygen. Conversely, the areas that are over-stimulated might have an excess of scarlet and need cooler colors. Furthers still, the sexual organs could finally turn purple, and thus advise their possessor to take mind. Whereas, areas of the body and mind with washed out, or muted colors, show a lack of sufficient vibrancy which indicates the reduced injection of color in the body.

When a healer understands the unique energetic vibration for each part of the body and the physical body as a whole, then they can use the aid of colors to achieve the same energetic vibration resonance. If, for example, they understand that the normal function of the certain part of the body can be restored by retuning its vibration, then the healing can be achieved.

Likewise, we can also tune into the energetic vibration we need by using our mind. This means that when we think about a certain color, then the vibration of our thoughts will also be raised to the vibration of that particular color. Then, when the vibration of our thoughts is raised to that level, it will then influence the overall vibration of our frame of mind. And, then, when the vibration of our thoughts and our frame of mind is at the same level, our physical body will then also begin to operate at that level. Which means that our thoughts, our frame of mind and our physical body will have the same energetic vibration. Then, when this happens, this overall vibration will affect the parts of the body and give them the instruction at which vibration they should operate. For example, if that energy was abnormal, its overall function will be restored based on the steady supply of proper vibration. Then, when they reach their proper vibration, this will reflect in their overall healing, and their function will return to normal.

18. Vortex energy healing

There are essentially two 'worlds' in existence, one is material (aka physical) and the other spiritual. These two worlds are in total, constant, and inseparable interaction with one another. The origin of the spiritual world is not physical. But the origin of the physical world is the spiritual world. This means that anything and everything in existence (everything material and beyond) wouldn't be possible without its spiritual counterpart. The spiritual world is what sustains the physical world and creates it into existence.

Every physical thing, or creature, in existence has its own spiritual counterpart in the spiritual realm. Everything has a spirit. Each spirit is in charge of its own creation. And the continued existence of everything in the physical world depends on this uninterrupted connection with its source (spirit). The spirit decides how a particular physical (material) thing should look, what it should do and what purpose it should serve. This means that whether or not any cell in the human body is turned on (created into material existence), or turned off (de-created from the material existence) is decided in accordance to the wishes and purposes of the spirit.

Suppose the spirit has chosen to discontinue from the physical body any number of cells. To do so it then has its sovereign prerogative to totally and completely withdraw itself from those cells. Doing so would then mean that those cells, which would then have no spirit energy whatsoever, are then completely gone (dematerialized), and have, so to speak, returned to the source. Likewise, if the spirit then chooses to add cells to the physical body, it can then add its spirit to the existing cells (create those new cells) so to speak, out of a thin air. Why out of a thin air? Because the spirit doesn't even need thin air. All it needs is its desire to create or de-create in order to fulfill its purposes.

When the spirit decides to create or de-create anything in the physical world the spirit follows natural procedures. One of those procedures is the interdimensional portals (doorways). The spirit uses these portals to connect to the physical world in order to create or de-create things. These portals are basically two types of vortices. One vortex creates anything the spirit wishes to send into existence. And the other is the vortex in the opposite direction, which then de-creates (sends that same energy in reverse, or back to its original source).

The easiest way to think of these two types of portals is in terms of two cone-shaped spirals (vortices). The vortex which moves clockwise and upwards to form a narrow cone at the top, takes the physical matter back into the spiritual (dissolves it back into the larger spirit). While the downward-pointing cone that moves counterclockwise sends the spirits energy back into the physical. This is how the spiritual energy can then become (create) anything which happens to suit its needs. To complicate this procedure just a little bit further, these two spirals meet at the area where the respective top and bottom of their cones meet to form what could really be called something of an hourglass shape. Another shape that is also resembles are the two triangles which form into a letter 'X'. Together these two corresponding vortices act as the gateway (interdimensional portal) which constantly sends the spirit (energy) in and out of existence.

In reality, the prototypes of these vortices are more common than you might think. Some even say that they represent an actual reality of everything and every energy which happens to travel in this world and the universe. A spiral, for example, can be observed when looking at such things as the storm like tornado. The spiral is responsible for the Carioles effect of the masses of clouds and air moving on the surface of the earth, and the way the water travels in the oceans. Pour out the water in the sink and you will see again that same spiral (funnel) effect. Our entire DNA structure is of course a spiral, the roots and branches of the trees, the vines, and many, many other things also have that same reminiscent spiral. None of this is coincidence.

Let's go back to the two corresponding conical vortices which form an 'X'. Whenever something comes out of existence in the physical world, its energy travels upward and clockwise up the vortex until it reaches its counterpart on the other side. Here, the pointed ends of both vortices meet. After reaching this 'bottleneck' the de-created physical matter still continues to travel upward and clockwise as it fully returns back (dematerializes) into its source. Conversely, if the spirit decides to manifest something into existence, it then takes its appropriate energy and sends it back down the spiral. This happens in a downward and counterclockwise motion.

It's like a spiral staircase in a tall round tower. The upper portion is the abode of the spirit and the lower is the abode of the physical world. Suppose then that someone decides to climb up those stairs from the bottom in a clockwise pattern in order to carry something to the very top. In that case they travel up the stairs in a clockwise direction. Then, when it's time to go back to the physical world then that someone goes back to the ground by traveling in a downward and counterclockwise direction.

19. Divine hand visualization

The divine has created everything in existence. This divine, or whatever name one may call it, is responsible for everything that goes on in the world. From the smallest atom to the largest space, nothing is outside its involvement. It is intimately involved in one's life and everything else; including healing. It provides the creative force, and looks after its creation to make sure that everything goes in accordance with its larger plan for the world. It imbues every human being and makes it part and parcel of that greater divine.

The divine energy doesn't just create something as one would when say, building a house, or baking a pie, or combining chemicals. It actually puts a part of itself in all that it creates. This means that we are not simply creatures. We are the rightful heirs and natural inheritors of this, so to speak, 'parental force'. The divine cares about its children. It cares about us all. We are a part of it and it looks after us as one would after their only child. And since we are the children of the divine, we are divine. Our divine nature is more than eager to help us create the achievement of anything we desire. And it gives us the energy to heal.

But there is such a thing as the existence of a "will" in the universe. And it means that the greater divine will never violate the sovereign will of the human, or go against it. If a person does not willingly volunteer the use of their divine energy to connect with the greater divine for healing, then the divine energy within them will simply have to stay put. On the other hand, if a person wills it that the divine within them connect with the greater divine for healing. Then in that case, and provided that that's indeed their will, their will to do so will be fully respected by the greater divine. If this level of cooperation is achieved, then the intelligence of the divine in that human and the intelligence of the greater divine will connect in order to work together in order to manifest the healing reality.

The divine in humans is always able, if they so choose, to have a total and uninterrupted access to the creative energy of the greater divine. This is because the divine energy of the human being is one and the same energy with the greater divine. They are actually inseparable from one another. But when the divine power of creativity travelled into the divine essence within each person, so likewise traveled the free will of the creator. With this creativity we can create anything. And since we can use our free will to create healing or illness, we likewise have a free will to live with the consequences of what we've chosen to create.

20. Forgiving

Whenever we fail to intentionally forgive someone for the perceived, or actual, past wrongs, we retain negative thoughts. Eventually, like begins to attract like and those dense thoughts create a physical illness. In order for us to heal we have to release the heavy thoughts. And without our permission they will not be released. If we fail to give ourselves the permission to let go of our negative thoughts then we will continue to punish ourselves with their heavy consequences. In this way the lack of forgiveness (aka the retention of dense thoughts) actually backfires on the unforgiving person by making them sick. When we stop punishing ourselves in this way and forgive ourselves we release the thoughts that caused us to punish ourselves. Our thought burden is lightened and we are free to heal.

To forgive it helps to understand what is being forgiven. A person like this can do this by taking a look at their life to find out what it is that causes them not to be able to forgive (let go of heavy thoughts). Perhaps its source was a painful or unpleasant confrontation they had with someone or something when they were a child, maybe someone broke their toy, or took something from them without their knowing, or maybe they felt their parents were unjust to them, etc. Whatever the situation they caused a person to retain self-victimizing thoughts. This is because the stored thoughts, if they are not properly released, continue to victimize people long after the event.

These heavy thoughts ultimately often find their expression in one's fears and phobias long after the event that caused them. They continue to manifest themselves in a person's life each time they happen to face similar situations. So, because a person didn't have the chance way-back-then to intentionally forgive (let go of those thoughts), those heavy thoughts continued to be stored in their frame of mind. These negative thoughts lowered the overall vibration of their frame of mind. Then, when the vibration of their overall frame of mind was lowered it then set a lower operational vibration for the rest of the body. Stress, tension and premature aging and the like are all lower physical vibration in which the negative vibration of those thoughts become manifest.

When the cause of an illness is indeed found to be caused by the lack of forgiveness, then a person has to forgive in order to heal. When they are able to do so with intention they can then allow themselves to release the heavy negative thoughts. If on the other hand, someone is somehow unwilling to release those negative thoughts (forgiving someone for causing them pain and discomfort) then those heavy thoughts will continue to lower the overall vibration of the physical body and result in illness. Only by addressing the source of an illness will a person find a lasting healing.

21. Regretlessness

We all have some regrets. Everyone has some things in their life they wished they did differently if they had a chance. For most people these regrets gradually move on and by and large do not noticeably affect their quality of life. While for some, these regrets can be so strong that they literally make them have negative physical feelings like panic, pain, anger. In that case, any healing will most certainly necessitate their letting go of the heavy negative thoughts (regrets).

The regrets come in many forms. Some have the regret of being unable to hold on to a particular job, or a regret at having their position terminated. Another person might regret that their life's love, or their life's purpose has not panned out as they hoped. Others might feel a sense of regret at never having been given their chance to succeed. Whatever one's reason for having regrets, it inevitably results in the continued abuse of their physical body with the lower (negative) physical vibrations. If a person is unable to let go of the thoughts of regrets they will continue to experience the vibration of those thoughts on their frame of mind. The persistent thought of lower vibration will cause the overall vibration of the frame of mind to be lowered. Like attracts like, so the low vibration of the frame of mind will then set a lower operational vibration for the rest of the body. Then, when the overall physical vibration is lowered, it will match the overall vibration of the physical illness. If not corrected, this will impact the overall physical health of their body.

143

22. The Universal Declaration:
I choose to be in balance

Everything that happens (or doesn't happen) to someone is ultimately based on their choice. And anything one intentionally chooses to happen to them will happen. The universe ultimately obeys this sovereign and divine choice which we have to create (accept) from the surroundings anything we desire. And everyone is ultimately in charge of their own their own world. To exercise one's divine and sovereign choice one has to first know that as a divine being they have the right to accept or refuse anything their world sends them. So, if they want to heal then all they have to do is make their choice intentionally known to the world that this is what they want. This sovereign and divine choice never goes away.

To understand how one's worldview is one's own to create with it what one wishes is to understand that one's world and everything that happens in it is only as real as it is real to a person who lives it and does the observing. This means that the reason our world appears real to us is because we believe that our world is as real as it gets. We convince ourselves that something is true or real by using our senses. These senses include the sense of hearing, seeing, smelling, touching, feeling, tasting, and so on and so forth. The information gathered by our senses is then compiled into pictures, concepts or ideas, whose reality we can then choose to accept, or deny. We use our senses to 'compile' our perception of reality in roughly the same way as when a chef combines various gathered ingredients in order to make up their version of the desired dish.

As our senses collect and process more and more information, we are then able to construct our own independent version of reality. This reality is how we view our whole world. For example, when one walks outside and feels cold and wet, and hears the raindrops fall, their mind uses this information to make up a picture which they can then accept as their reality. This choice also means that if a different person also happens to walk outside and receive the same information, their senses may or may not cause them to construct a similar version of reality. That would be based on individual choice (aka free will). So, whereas one group of people comes out and feels cold and wet, it's also probable that the other group of people might see a totally different reality. These people might take the same, seemingly undisputed sensory data and interpret it in their own way. They might for example actually ignore the cold and continue to feel warm, because they won't feel the cold in the same way. Or, they might consider the rain just a sprinkle.

If we have a sovereign and divine choice to create our own version of reality based on the input we derive from our senses, doesn't it also mean that we can also change our perception of reality by changing how we interpret our sensory input? If we can do that, then we can surely change our own version of reality. This means that instead of just choosing to adjust our sensory data to our perceived reality, we can actually change our current version of perceived reality by changing how we interpret our sensory data. But before we can exchange one reality for another, we have to accept that the reality we want to experience is actually real. For example, if we want to experience the reality of healing, then we have to accept that that reality is real. If we can accept that our choice is real, then the rest of the world will have to respect this sovereign and divine choice and adjust itself in accordance with our newly accepted version of reality.

In order for our reality to begin to make its appropriate adjustments and reinforce our newly accepted version of reality, all we have to do then is to then intentionally choose to experience it. For example, if an ill person accepts the reality that they are healing, they can then make that choice intentionally known to the rest of their world. If that choice happens to be strong, the resulting reality will be created. Their choice to experience that reality will cause their sensory input to adjust (change) to conform to their reality. As soon as the choice is intentionally made, their health will have no other choice but to move in the direction of their accepted reality. Conversely, if one intentionally chooses not to accept their healing as real, and make that sovereign and divine request clearly known, then truly there is absolutely no force in the world to prove to them that it isn't so.

23. Believing

A wise healer clearly understands that every illness originates with the frame of mind (aka human consciousness). And how a person's frame of mind operates is determined by their belief. This means that a wise healer begins the restoration of their patient's health with the restoration of their patient's faith in the healer's medicine. You noticed here the word 'healer' as opposed to the 'medical doctor'. That is because knowing medicine is unlike having the wisdom of healing. One can be full of knowledge and have no track record of healing.

A wise healer understands that in themselves any medicines and medical treatments are powerless. And that those treatments are only as strong as a patient's faith in them. Some people can still fall ill and remain ill even with the best available medicine. So, at the beginning of the healing process a healer tries to understand the condition of a person's frame of mind and how it caused an illness. This is done by probing the degree of their patient's faith in the healer's medicine. Then when they get a good idea of the kind of beliefs that make up their patient's frame of mind, a healer then proceeds to tailor their conversation to the patient, and adjust their healing treatment to best compliment their patient's beliefs.

Very rarely would a genuine healer seek to change their patient's beliefs outright and thereby their frame of mind.

Often they simply begin their patient's healing by restoring their faith in their own ability to heal with the healer's medicines. If done very skillfully, a patient will never realize what actually happened. Instead, they'll start to attribute their healing to the medical treatment alone. Not to their restored belief in a healer's medicine.

A different thinking goes through the mind of a healer than that of a patient. While a patient places their trust (faith) in their healer's medicine, a healer only uses the medicine as a tool to help their patient believe that they can heal and that they are healing. Unlike a patient, a healer never regards the medicine as the actual thing that healed their patient. A healer never loses the sight that it is the inner power within their patient that ultimately did the actual healing. Not the medicine. A wise healer is able to achieve this degree of mastery, because they do not look at healing as a means to get praises and recognition, or to prove the effectiveness of their medicine. Looking for rewards is not the same as harnessing the innate power within the patient to be healthy.

Another important thing that happens with a wise healer is that they always make sure not to intentionally delude their patient. A patient is not to end up in the situation where they end up not healing and then blaming everything on the medicine (or the pill) that they took. A healer knows better than to carelessly encourage their patient to place all their faith and responsibility for healing on a 'magical pill'. Healing is not about illusions. Healing is not about placing a blind faith in anything. And a wise healer knows that only the patient has the power to heal themselves. Their faith in that ability to be healthy must be restored. And a wise healer encourages their patient to do what only they can: to heal themselves.

Each of us has a potential to become a healer of others, but before we heal others of the same illnesses, we must first learn to heal a patient within ourselves. A wise healer can only show us the way and give us knowledge. But only we have the ability to take that knowledge and convert it into wisdom. When we apply that knowledge enough times we'll wise up, and a wise healer within us will heal ourselves.

24. Staying positive

A physical illness in itself is neither good nor evil. And ultimately it's neither positive nor negative. It's what each person ultimately makes of it. An illness appears bad and evil because of what we make out of that experience. But oftentimes it isn't an illness that's evil, it's our heavy (negative) thoughts. This is because our thoughts create our reality. And a lot of our illnesses are manifested by negative thoughts.

Physical illness is ultimately just a thought form (a thought) which is neither good nor evil. If our thoughts are full of the thought forms of illness and absence of healing, then those thoughts determine our reality. And ultimately determine how those thoughts are manifested in the reality of our physical body.

Each thought is also positive or negative relative to the observer. Which is another way of saying a higher vibration and a lower vibration. Every thought then, has its own vibration. Basically, some thoughts have a higher vibration and some thoughts have a lower vibration. You can usually tell that by how those thoughts make you feel. Whether they make you feel elevated (light) or depressed (weighed down). For example, anger, hatred and fear are the thoughts of lower vibration because they cause the physical body to feel depressed. While the thoughts of peace and love are considered to be the thoughts of higher vibration because they cause the physical body to feel elated.

When a person feels negative a lot of the times this means that their thoughts are dominated by negative (lower vibration) thoughts. And since like attracts like, eventually this could result in the attraction of the physical illness (lower vibration) thought form to the body. Then, when the heavy thought form starts to influence the overall vibration of their frame of mind, it will then match the lower vibration of the physical illness. This will cause the feeling of illness to become manifested in a physical form. And they will feel ill.

This basic process of manifesting the reality of the physical illness goes like this. At first a person's overall vibration has to be lowered to match the lower vibration of an illness. In order to do this a person has to lower the overall vibration of their physical body to match the overall vibration of the physical illness. This is achieved by lowering the overall vibration of their frame of mind. Meanwhile, the lowering of the overall vibration of their frame of mind is achieved by lowering the overall quality of their thoughts. Then, when the overall vibration of their thoughts, their frame of mind, and their physical body reaches the same vibration as the physical illness it will then cause their physical body to operate at that vibration. Then, in response to operating at that heavy vibration their physical body will feel physically ill.

If a person wants to attract more healing and manifest physical health in their body, they have to take the opposite route. In that case a person has to raise their overall vibration to more closely match the higher vibration of the healing they desire. To do this they first have to increase the overall vibration of their thoughts. They have to let go of the heavy thought forms (like anger, hatred, and fear) which weigh them down, and accept lighter vibration thought forms. That's because the overall vibration of the frame of mind is determined by the overall vibration of the thought vibration at which it operates. A basic way to lighten the load is to keep track of how each thought makes them feel. If for example, a specific thought makes them tense up and become uncomfortable, then they will be able to tell if that thought is worth keeping.

Once a person has raised the vibration of their thought forms they can then raise the vibration of their overall frame of mind. Like attracts like. So, if for example their frame of mind is nourished by positive thoughts, then that will mean that the overall vibration of their frame of mind will likewise be increased. Then, when the frame of mind reaches a similar higher vibration, then it will set the overall operational vibration of the rest of their physical body. Then, when the vibration of the thoughts, the frame of mind and the physical body all reach the same higher level, then the thought cycle will be completed and their overall physical body will operate at a higher vibration. Then, when their overall vibration reaches a positive level, it will then match the similar higher vibrations of the healing. Meanwhile, the lower vibration of the illness thought form will not have a matching physical vibration, and therefore won't be further manifested in the physical body.

25. Making your intent

Without the intent the thought manifestation process wouldn't be possible. And in order for a thought to be manifested in the physical world, it needs an intent.

Every thought is a vibration, and not all thoughts (thought forms) that enter the frame of mind ultimately become manifested in the physical world. Likewise, not every thought vibration can end up being materialized in the physical world. What bridges the gap between the vibration of the thought form and the corresponding vibration of created physical object is the intent for it to happen. If there is no intent, then the vibration of the thought form does not turn into a vibration of a material object. On the other hand, once the intention is applied to manifest a thought form into a physical object (or a physical action), a person then has to live with the consequences of every part of what they intended to do. This is why even the smallest intent to do something has far-reaching consequences.

Once a person has an intent to do something (manifest the thought vibration into a physical vibration), they can then manifest that object into the physical world. This means that if a person has a thought that they want to heal, they can then apply their intent to that thought form and manifest that thought of healing in their physical body. For example, if a person has a desire (a thought form) to raise the overall vibration of their physical body in order to heal, they can begin this by using their intent to raise the vibration of their thought forms. If they don't have the intent to raise the vibration of their thoughts, then that thought will not be ultimately manifested into their physical body. If they have the intent to raise the vibration of their thoughts to match the higher vibration of healing, then the vibration of their frame of mind will likewise be raised.

As long as they have the intent to raise the vibration of their thoughts then the vibration of their thoughts will be raised. By applying an intent to those thoughts, they will be able to focus and concentrate on being careful what thoughts enter their frame of mind. If they have the intent to have their frame of mind be nourished by positive higher vibration thoughts, then the overall vibration of their frame of mind will also be raised to that level. Then once their frame of mind and their thoughts operate at the same vibration level, it will only be a matter of time before their frame of mind will set the overall operational vibration rate for their physical body. Then, once the thought cycle is complete and their thoughts, their frame of mind and their physical body have a matching vibration, then the overall higher vibration of their physical body will match with the higher vibration of healing. Then, when their vibration is the same as the vibration of the healing, their physical body will attract healing. Meanwhile, the vibration of illness will be too low and won't match their overall vibration.

26. Being creative

To create something means to manifest something. And the process of manifestation is ultimately a process of converting (materializing) the vibration of a thought into a physical object. This is because everything is manifested from a thought and a thought precedes the manifestation of the physical form. When the thought (aka thought form) becomes manifested in the physical object the vibration of that object is similar to its original thought. The only difference, which is ultimately not even a difference at all, is that one thought is materialized in the physical object while the other is not. Additionally, since the vibration of the thought form and the physical object is the same, they are ultimately the same physical object and a thought form. And the physical objects that have the same vibration are the same objects. And anything that vibrates at the same rate as something else becomes the same physical object.

At the beginning of the manifestation process is an idea. This initial idea is also called a thought or a thought form, and it is a key step in the physical manifestation process. Basically, once there is a thought form, this thought form then finds its way into a person's frame of mind. Once there, the vibration of that thought form begins to set the overall operational vibration rate of the frame of mind. This happens because the objects that vibrate at the same rate become the same object. Then, when the overall vibration of the frame of mind reaches the same rate as the vibration of the original thought form, they are said to have a matching vibration. Then, once the vibration of the thought form and the frame of mind is the same, then the vibration of the frame of mind sets the operational vibration for the rest of the physical body. Then, once the vibration of the thought form, the frame of mind and the physical body reach the same level, then that thought form becomes materialized in the physical body. This is the point where the thought form cycle is complete.

In a broader explanation of the physical manifestation process things aren't as simple. The first major difference is that many of the physical objects are not made up of a single vibration. And their overall vibration is made up of many other vibrations. This is why you can't simply think 'million dollars' and then manifest it into your reality. The million dollars is made up of many additional thought vibrations that are essential to its fuller manifestation. So, thinking a number like a million dollars isn't a broader story. There's also the ink, the paper, or an electronic account, and countless other thought vibrations that go along with that. Another example would be the construction of a building. Again, here the overall vibration of the building is made up of many other vibrations. The window glass has a different vibration, so does the steel and wood trusses, stones, concrete, wiring, etc. This means that in order to have the idea of a building be manifested in the physical reality, the thought vibrations of all those building components must be obtained separately and then put together. No thought form is to be overlooked if that building is to be built. Even the separate thought form vibrations which make up a single nail must be attained. The vibration of everything you want to be manifested in your physical reality must be obtained.

Another important difference to consider in the explanation of a thought manifestation process is that we create things in the universe out of the universal matter. The universal matter is essentially a reflection of the latent thought form vibrations and their infinite combinations. And it is up to us to take those physically manifested thought form vibrations and combine (reconstitute) them into the overall vibrations of what we want. In this way the world serves as the kind of repository of all of the physically manifested vibrations of various thought forms. In this process, if we want to physically manifest (create) our particular thought form, we use the vibration of that thought form to change the overall vibration of our frame of mind to that level. We then physically manifest that vibration by looking for the presence of that matching vibration in the physical forms. Eventually, we find (attract) the physical object(s) whose cumulative vibration matches the overall vibration of our original thought form. To finish our final product we might also have to trim or increase the overall vibration of that physical object, or recombine it with some other object to make it ultimately match our desired vibration. In this way we are creating (manifesting) our final physical product into reality.

In order to create our desired level of health we don't have to create another physical body. The one we've got will do just fine. All we need to do to heal is raise the overall physical vibration of our body in order to match the vibration of health. Then, when the vibration of our physical body operates at a different rate, the body's overall vibration will be recombined (reconstituted) to match that vibration. Conversely, if our choice is to lower our overall vibration, then we just use lower thought forms to reconstitute the overall vibration of our physical body to operate at a lower level.

For this manifestation to work means we have to have an idea of what it is that we want to create. Once we have that idea, we can then use its thought vibration as a reference while we look for it in the existing repository of physical objects. Or, if necessary, to recombine the other existing objects (vibrations) to match the vibration level of our original thought form. In this way, we can make ourselves healthier by understanding what the vibration of that physical health is in order to raise our overall physical vibration to match that level. Then, once we become familiar with what that vibration (idea) is we can then refer to it while we raise the overall vibration of our physical bodies.

27. The last thought of the day

Every thought we have is ultimately the same. And the kind of thoughts we have in our mind is determined by whether or not the overall vibration of those thoughts happens to match the overall vibration of our frame of mind. If the overall vibration of the thoughts (thought forms) matches the overall vibration of the frame of mind, then they are accepted. If not, they are repelled. And in this way there's a constant interaction between the two, because the vibration of the thought forms sets the overall vibration of the frame of mind. And the vibration of the frame of mind determines what thoughts it chooses to accept or repel.

The overall vibration of the physical body is also determined by the overall vibration of the frame of mind. And once the overall vibration of the frame of mind is set by the overall vibration of its thought forms, it can then set the operational vibration for the rest of the physical body. So that ultimately, how the physical body operates is determined by the kind of thoughts that are accepted or repelled by the frame of mind. In this way some experience the physical vibration of an illness and some experience the physical vibration of the healing.

Since every thought in the frame of mind is ultimately the same, this means that these thoughts all have something in common. They all share a common vibration. This can be understood as an object (or a thought) vibration that has some aspects of it in common with all of the other objects (thought vibrations). You can use any example to experiment with this concept, or use any common object as a reference. Some objects, have roundness (or circles) in common. While some objects (thoughts) have squares and triangles etc. All this means is that all these objects (thought forms) share similar vibrations. And the kind of thought forms that are present in our frame of mind at a given moment is determined by whether or not the vibration of those thoughts matches the overall vibration of our frame of mind. The easiest way to understand this is that when someone is hungry they tend to fixate more on food and see things that look like foods. If you ever shopped on a hungry stomach, you get the idea.

The thought of a physical illness or healing essentially operates in the same way as any other thoughts. The thoughts of illness attract other thoughts of illness because of the matching thought vibrations. And the thoughts of the healing attract other thoughts of the healing because of the matching vibrations. Ultimately, whether a person has the thoughts of the physical illness or a physical healing, those thought vibrations become manifested in the overall vibration of their physical body. Then, when their overall vibration reaches the same vibration as the thought of either illness or healing, their physical body ends up either feeling ill or healthy.

When we understand how the vibration of our positive (healing) or negative (illness) thoughts sets the overall vibration of the rest of our physical body, we can then be more aware about what thought forms we choose to accept or repel from our frame of mind. If, for example, we want our physical body to reach the vibration of healing, then we can make sure that our frame of mind is predominated by the positive thoughts which we want to manifest into reality. It's all based on the thought choices we choose to make.

When you go to sleep you have the opportunity to determine at what vibration you want your physical body to operate. If your choice is to raise the overall vibration of your physical body, then take care that your last thought of the day is centered on healing and positive thoughts. Beware, that if you neglect this and let your mind spiral out of control with more and more thoughts of the same illness and negativity, this will lower the overall vibration of your frame of mind. These thoughts will pull down the vibration of your frame of mind, and with it the overall vibration of the rest of your body. These are not the best consequences if your present goal is to achieve healing. So, try to relax and think positive.